The clinical applications of human gene therapy have been particularly fruitful in oncology, and in the last two decades there has been explosive growth in understanding of the genetic lesions leading to neoplasia. This volume in the series *Cancer: Clinical Science in Practice* reviews progress in the basic and clinical science of gene therapy in oncology, and looks forward to future developments. It considers what has worked and what has not in the fast-evolving field of gene therapy, drawing on laboratory studies and clinical trials, including the ground-breaking work of the contributors themselves. Elucidation of fundamental genetic differences between normal and tumor cells, and identification of tumor-specific DNA sequences are being exploited in novel therapies by a number of targeting strategies outlined here.

Up-to-date and authoritative, volumes in this series are intended for a wide audience of clinicians and researchers with an interest in the application of biomedical science to the understanding and management of cancer.

T0321604

GENE THERAPY IN THE TREATMENT OF CANCER:
PROGRESS AND PROSPECTS

CANCER: CLINICAL SCIENCE IN PRACTICE

General Editor
Professor Karol Sikora
Department of Clinical Oncology
Royal Postgraduate Medical School
Hammersmith Hospital, London

A series of authoritative review volumes intended for a wide audience of clinicians and researchers with an interest in the application of biomedical science to the understanding and management of cancer.

Also in this series
Drug Resistance in the Treatment of Cancer
ISBN 0 521 473217
Edited by Herbert M. Pinedo and Giuseppe Giaccone

Tumor Immunology: Immunotherapy and cancer vaccines
ISBN 0 521 427 377
Edited by A. G. Dalgleish and M. J. Browning

Cell Therapy
ISBN 0 521 473152
Edited by George Morstyn and William P. Sheridan

Molecular Endocrinology of Cancer
ISBN 0 521 473670
Edited by Jonathan Waxman

GENE THERAPY IN THE TREATMENT OF CANCER

Progress and Prospects

Edited by
BRIAN E. HUBER
Glaxo Wellcome Company, North Carolina, USA
and
IAN MAGRATH
National Cancer Institute, Bethesda, Maryland, USA

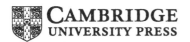

CAMBRIDGE
UNIVERSITY PRESS

CAMBRIDGE UNIVERSITY PRESS
Cambridge, New York, Melbourne, Madrid, Cape Town, Singapore, São Paulo

Cambridge University Press
The Edinburgh Building, Cambridge CB2 2RU, UK

Published in the United States of America by Cambridge University Press, New York

www.cambridge.org
Information on this title: www.cambridge.org/9780521444361

First published 1998
This digitally printed first paperback version 2006

A catalogue record for this publication is available from the British Library

ISBN-13 978-0-521-44436-1 hardback
ISBN-10 0-521-44436-5 hardback

ISBN-13 978-0-521-03351-0 paperback
ISBN-10 0-521-03351-9 paperback

Contents

Contents

Contributors

Kishor Bhatia
Section of Lymphoma Biology, National Cancer Institute, National Institutes of Health, 9000 Rockville Pike, Bethesda, Maryland 20892, USA

Alfred E. Chang
Department of Surgery, University of Michigan Medical Center, 1500 East Medical Center Drive, Ann Arbor, Michigan 48109, USA

J. Patrick Condreay
Glaxo Wellcome Company, Research Triangle Park, North Carolina 27709, USA

Patrick J. Geraghty
Department of Surgery, University of Michigan Medical Center, 1150 West Medical Center Drive, Ann Arbor, Michigan 48109, USA

Brian E. Huber
Director, Division of Pharmacology, Glaxo Wellcome Company, Research Triangle Park, North Carolina 27709, USA

Kanak Iyer
Medicine Branch, National Cancer Institute, National Institutes of Health, 9000 Rockville Pike, Bethesda, Maryland 20892, USA

John C. Krauss
The Cleveland Clinic Foundation, 9500 Euclid Avenue, Cleveland, Ohio 44195, USA

Ian Magrath
Section of Lymphoma Biology, National Institutes of Health, 9000 Rockville Pike, Bethesda, Maryland 20892, USA

James J. Mulé
*Department of Surgery and Bone Marrow Transplant Program, University
of Michigan Medical Center, 1150 West Medical Center Drive, Ann Arbor,
Michigan 48109, USA*

Leonard M. Neckers
*Medicine Branch, National Cancer Institute, National Institutes of Health,
9000 Rockville Pike, Bethesda, Maryland 20892, USA*

Cynthia A. Richards
*Department of Cancer Biology, Glaxo Wellcome Company, Research Triangle
Park, North Carolina 27709, USA*

Jack A. Roth
*Department of Thoracic and Cardiovascular Surgery, The University of Texas,
M.D. Anderson Cancer Center, Houston, Texas 77030, USA*

Prem Seth
*Medical Breast Cancer Section, Medicine Branch, National Cancer Institute,
National Institutes of Health, 9000 Rockville Pike, Bethesda, Maryland 20892,
USA*

Suyu Shu
*Department of Surgery, University of Michigan Medical Center, 1500 East
Medical Center Drive, Ann Arbor, Michigan 48109, USA*

Preface

Cancer is now the biggest target disease for gene therapy protocols worldwide. Despite significant advances in the treatment of cancer in the last two decades, most tumors remain resistant to all current treatment modalities – surgery, radiotherapy, chemotherapy, and biotherapy. Local methods such as surgery and radiotherapy are often only effective in the absence of metastatic disease. Despite tremendous effort over the last fifty years, only a very small proportion of human cancers are cured by chemotherapy.

Gene-based therapy is a novel therapeutic approach to treating cancer which has been made possible only by recent and remarkable progress in our understanding of the molecular biology of cancer. Gene therapy can be described as the transfer to human cells and the expression of genetic material for a therapeutic purpose. Currently there are over two hundred gene therapy protocols active worldwide specifically aimed at single gene defects such as cystic fibrosis and a growing number of cancers. This book outlines the diverse approaches being attempted to develop effective future cancer therapies.

The last decade has seen dramatic advances in our understanding of the mechanisms involved in the control of cell growth and their deregulation in cancer. Certain classes of genes encode proteins that play distinct roles in the processing of signals from the outside of the cell to the nucleus. Any changes to the delicate system of control by these oncogenes or tumor suppressor genes may result in the formation of cancer. It is becoming increasingly clear that pre-existing genetic factors and environmental events combine to cause the series of molecular changes that are necessary for tumor formation. Elucidation of fundamental genetic differences between normal and tumor cells and identification of tumor-specific DNA sequences are being exploited in novel therapies by a number of targeting strategies outlined here.

Karol Sikora

1

Introduction: gene therapy approaches to cancer

BRIAN E. HUBER

It is interesting to reflect back on the literature written between 1980 and 1987 regarding the prospects and anticipated first applications of human gene therapy. What were predicted with a fair degree of accuracy were the specific gene transfer technologies that would first be utilized in the initial human gene therapy protocols: liposomal-mediated gene transfer and gene transfer via replication-defective retroviral and adenoviral vectors. The vast majority of human gene transfer protocols to date have used these transfer technologies. However, it was not originally anticipated that naked DNA would be efficacious in certain specific tissues, such as muscle, for gene transfer and expression.

What were neither anticipated nor predicted with any degree of accuracy were the target diseases for the initial human gene therapy protocols. These were originally predicted to be primarily monogenetic diseases, some of which are listed in Table 1.1. However, although the very first pioneering human gene therapy protocol, performed on September 14, 1990, was for correction of adenosine deaminase deficiency disease – a milestone event in the continual evolution of modern medicine – this prediction has proved to be incorrect. Instead, reflecting back over the last few years, it is clear that most of the initial applications have been in the oncology area, and it is interesting to examine the evolution of human gene therapy over this period.

Figure 1.1 illustrates the increase in the number of human gene therapy protocols approved by the Recombinant DNA Advisory Committee (RAC) that has taken place over the last few years in the United States – a total of 132 protocols by November 1996. It is apparent that there was an almost yearly exponential increase in the number of protocols submitted and approved up to 1995, but that the rate of submissions and approvals significantly slowed after that. This is due to a decline in the number of protocols submitted for approval rather than to a decrease in the success rate in the approval process

1

Table 1.1. *Monogenetic diseases anticipated to be the initial target diseases for the application of human gene therapy*

Adenosine deaminase deficiency
Purine nucleoside phosphorylase deficiency
Hypoxanthine–guanine phosphoribosyltransferase deficiency
Factor VIII deficiency
Factor IX deficiency
Sickle cell anemia
β-Thalassemia
Ornithine transcarbamylase deficiency
Argininosuccinate synthetase deficiency
α1-Antitrypsine deficiency
Glucocerebrosidase deficiency

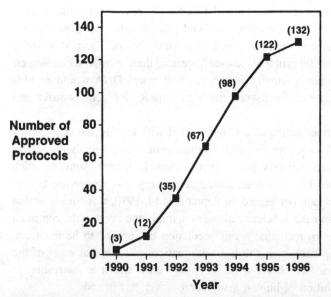

Fig. 1.1. Approved gene therapy protocols in the USA. The number of approvals was determined based on summation of Review level 1 through Review level 4 approvals. Approvals are classified as follows.
Review level 1: full RAC review + NIH Director approval + FDA Investigational New Drug (IND) approval. *Review level 2:* accelerated RAC review + NIH Office of Recombinant DNA activities (ORDA) approval + FDA IND approval. *Review level 3:* sole FDA review (simultaneous submission to NIH (ORDA) for the purpose of data monitoring and adverse event reporting. *Review level 4:* sole FDA review (submission to NIH (ORDA) not required). (For reference see: dwknorr/protocol/ protocol.new/October9,1996 on the HHS/NIH/RAC home page.)

Table 1.2. *Gene-transfer techniques and methodology for approved protocols in the United States*

Gene-transfer technique
  80 Ex-vivo gene transfer
  52 In-vivo gene transfer

Gene-transfer method
  87 Retroviral vectors
  16 Adenoviral vectors
  2 adeno-associated viral vectors
  1 Pox vector
  20 Cationic liposomes
  4 Plasmid DNA
  1 Particle mediated
  1 Vaccinia virus vector

itself. It is anticipated that the number of submissions and approvals during the remainder of this decade will be somewhat lower than that in the first half of the decade. Approximately 40 human gene therapy protocols have been approved in Europe during the same period.

Due both to safety concerns and to the limitations of gene-transfer technology, the first human gene therapy protocols predominantly involved ex-vivo gene-transfer techniques (Table 1.2). However, as confidence in safety has increased, so has the number of approvals for protocols involving in-vivo gene transfer. As predicted, the gene-transfer methodology that has predominated in the initial protocols has involved the use of replication-deficient viral vectors and cationic liposomes, despite the many significant limitations associated with retroviral vectors (Table 1.1).

In the United States, almost 1000 patients have participated in in-vivo or ex-vivo gene therapy protocols at the time of writing. The toxicities that have been reported to date have been related either to physiologic responses to expression of the transgenes or to acute toxicities associated with the delivery vectors themselves. There have been no reports of viral vector recombination or permanent toxicities due to transgene integration.

Table 1.3 illustrates the therapeutic areas in which gene therapy protocols have been approved in the United States and Europe. The vast majority of the 132 approved protocols in the US has been for oncology indications (approximately 73%), as have approximately 80% of those in Europe.

Why has the oncology field dominated the initial clinical development of human gene therapy? Table 1.4 lists some of the reasons, the main one

Table 1.3. *Therapeutic areas for approved gene therapy*
protocols

Current roster of protocols approved by RAC (1996)	
Total gene-marking protocols	29
Total gene therapy protocols	132
Cancer	96
Genetic deficiency diseases	21
AIDS	12
Vascular diseases	2
Rheumatoid arthritis	1
Current roster of protocols approved in Europe (1996)	
Total gene therapy protocols	40
Cancer	32
Cystic fibrosis	5
Adenosine deaminase deficiency (ADA)	3

Table 1.4. *Gene therapy targeted to cancer*

1. Unmet medical need
2. Life-threatening disease
3. Very large, dispersed patient population
4. Commercially viable
5. Molecular mechanisms in pathophysiology
6. Multiple diseases
   Multiple mechanisms

concerning the current state of efficacy, or lack thereof, of conventional cancer treatments. There is a tremendous unmet medical need for new, innovative and unconventional approaches to cancer treatment, any which are developed being embraced by patients, clinicians and regulatory authorities. In most situations, clinicians are dealing with a life-threatening disease that requires the making of bold decisions about experimental therapeutic approaches. The cost (safety/toxicity)/benefit (potential cure or palliation) ratio is shifted toward experimental therapies since conventional therapies usually fail in this life-threatening situation.

The cancer patient population is large and dispersed throughout the world, permitting experimental clinical trials in the developed world. This fact, coupled with the significant unmet medical need in the developed world, has attracted both small biotechnology companies and large pharmaceutical companies to focus on this area. In addition, there has been a tremendous increase in understanding of the molecular etiology of neoplastic disease over the last 15 years. Many causative and contributing genetic lesions have been identified for a variety of neoplasms, including the expression of oncogenes, the loss of function of tumor suppressor genes, and acquisition of resistance to chemotherapy through altered gene expression. This has given unique insights into the molecular pathophysiology of the disease, which has fostered extremely rational gene therapy approaches. Cancer has also dominated the initial clinical development of gene therapy due to its nature. Neoplastic disease is not one disease resulting from the same genetic lesions producing similar pathologic phenotypes. Rather, it may be considered to be 150 to 200 different neoplastic or paraneoplastic diseases, with different genetic lesions resulting in different phenotypic characteristics. This lends itself to a variety of different approaches and techniques depending on the particular tumor type. Hence, multiple approaches to multiple tumor types can be investigated simultaneously. Chapter 2 of this book describes the types of genetic lesions that are thought to play a causative role in cancer formation and, based on that knowledge, the development of transformation-specific therapy. A critical element in successful transformation-specific theory is the delivery system, whereby a therapeutic agent is introduced into the target tissue. A number of delivery systems (vectors) are described in Chapter 3.

As stated above, gene therapy can be experimentally and clinically utilized in a multitude of novel and diverse approaches to the treatment of cancer. Figure 1.2 illustrates some of these approaches, which can be separated into two broad categories based on the target cell of the genetic manipulation: either the tumor cells themselves or normal, noncancerous cells.

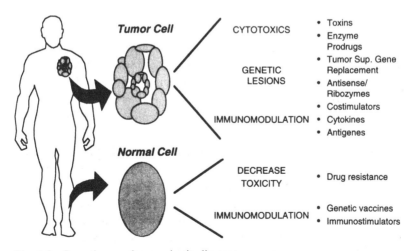

Fig. 1.2. Gene therapy for neoplastic diseases.

The tumor cell as the gene-transfer target cell

There has been proposed a multitude of gene therapy approaches that target the tumor cell as the cell that is genetically manipulated. One approach is to transfer into the tumor cells, genes which encode direct-acting toxins, such as Pseudomonas B toxin, expression of which will theoretically kill the tumor cell. The major concern with this approach is the lack of control and safety associated with overexpression or inappropriate expression of the toxin gene. For this reason, transfer and expression of genes encoding direct-acting and potent toxins have not been explored clinically. Another way to generate a cytotoxic molecule is to transfer a gene that encodes a prodrug-activation enzyme. This is a two-phase approach, which may have greater safety and control associated with it. The prodrug-activating enzyme will have no intrinsic toxicity associated with its expression. However, the presence of the enzyme results in conversion of nontoxic prodrugs into cytotoxic agents within the tumor cells but not in normal cells which lack the enzyme. Application of this approach is covered in Chapter 4.

Another approach that targets the tumor mass for gene transfer is the delivery of genes whose expression is directed specifically at interfering with the genetic aberrations that cause the transformation process. For example, the tumor mass can be targeted with genes that encode dominant negative proteins, antisense molecules, or ribozymes that inhibit specific oncogenes. Alternatively, the tumor mass can be targeted with genes that encode functional tumor suppressor genes, such as *p53*, to restore the function lost through mutational events. The approach of targeting tumor cells with genes that either inactivate oncogenes or restore the function of tumor suppressor genes is covered in Chapter 5.

Another approach to targeting the tumor mass is the delivery of genes expressing immunostimulators. The basis of this approach is that normally an intact, functioning immune system can effectively survey, identify, and eliminate neoplastic cells. However, in relatively rare instances, the immune system cannot recognize or is unable to eliminate these transformed cells, which results in cancer. Neoplastic cells have certain properties that may hinder the immune system from recognizing and eliminating them. For example, certain tumor cells have a decrease in expression of the major histocompatibility complex, which is essential for displaying and presenting tumor-associated antigens to cells of the immune system. In addition, tumor cells can express specific factors that may block or inhibit the cascade of events necessary for a robust cytotoxic T lymphocyte response (CTL), which is required for immunologic elimination of the tumor mass.

There have been a number of related approaches attempting to transfer into the tumor mass genes which encode factors that may increase the recognition of the tumor by the immune system or the robustness of the immune system's overall response. These approaches are described in Chapters 6 and 7.

The normal cell as the gene-transfer target cell

The tumor mass does not have to be the target for gene transfer. Rather, in some approaches, normal cells may be the target for genetic manipulation. One example of this involves the delivery of drug-resistance genes to normal cells that are the site of dose-limiting toxicity for specific conventional chemotherapy. Particularly relevant targets may be bone marrow, lung, cardiac tissue, and liver. Genes that encode either the multidrug resistance P-glycoprotein or very specific drug detoxification enzymes may be relevant. These approaches are discussed in Chapter 4.

Another approach targeting normal cells is the genetic manipulation of cells of the immune system, such as CTL, tumor-infiltrating lymphocytes (TIL), or hematopoietic stem cells. The very first gene-transfer experiments were performed to assess the viability, targeting, and half-life of TIL cells. Chapter 7 deals with the use of cytokine genes, and with genes encoding the

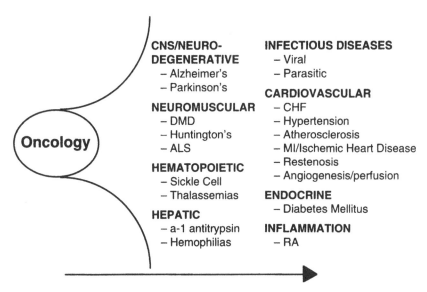

Fig. 1.3. Advancement of gene therapy into other therapeutic areas. CHF, chronic heart failure; MI, myocardial infarction; RA, rheumatoid arthritis; DMD, Duchenne's muscular dystrophy; ALS, amyotrophic lateral sclerosis.

T cell receptor(s), chemokine, and chemokine receptors. The clinical status of these approaches is summarized in Chapters 7 and 9.

Finally, Chapter 10 provides some practical considerations for the production and safety testing of gene-transfer vectors commonly used in human gene therapy protocols.

Although this book deals specifically with the applications of gene therapy in oncology, the pioneering and ground-breaking advances of gene therapy in oncology will certainly have positive spin-offs in other therapeutic areas (Figure 1.3).

2

Principles of transformation-directed cancer therapy

IAN MAGRATH AND KISHOR BHATIA

Introduction

While approximately half of all patients with cancer can be cured, either by locoregional therapy (surgery or radiation) or by systemic chemotherapy, this success is not gained without a price – that of toxicity to normal tissues, either during treatment or afterwards. Prominent among the late effects of treatment is the development of second malignancies, for radiation and chemotherapy are both carcinogenic (Boice, 1988; Boffetta and Kaldor, 1994). The protean toxic manifestations of cancer therapy arise because of the lack of selectivity of present treatment approaches, a shortcoming that is hardly surprising when it is considered that the therapeutic effects of radiation and chemotherapy were first recognized, and have subsequently been enhanced, almost entirely as a consequence of empirical observations. Thus, all new approaches to cancer treatment are directed towards improving the therapeutic index, i.e., decreasing toxicity while achieving similar, or preferably better, tumor cell kill. While empirical clinical trials remain the mainstay of research directed towards the improvement of therapeutic results, it seems probable that optimal therapeutic indices, in which curative therapy is associated with minimal toxicity (i.e., tumor-specific therapy), will only be achieved by the identification of major biological differences between neoplastic cells and their normal counterparts that can be exploited therapeutically (i.e., the identification of an 'Achilles heel' in the tumor cell). In the last two decades, there has been explosive growth in our understanding of the genetic lesions that lead to the deregulated growth and differentiation of neoplastic cells, and the recognition that the very lesions that cause cancer are, by definition, unique to the tumor cells. Since these primary genetic derangements are essential to the cell's neoplastic behavior, the most selective approaches to therapy are likely to be those directed towards transformation-specific molecular abnormalities.

This chapter briefly surveys the tumor-specific targets that result from the genetic changes that give rise to cancer, and describes some of the approaches that can be considered in attempting to exploit them therapeutically.

Transformation-specific targets for cancer therapy

The earliest attempts to develop tumor-specific therapy were, not surprisingly, based on the assumption that there should be antigenic differences between cancer cells and normal cells (Luders et al., 1985; Suter et al., 1985). In animal tumors this is often the case, and considerable success has been achieved with immunotherapeutic approaches based on the interaction of antibody or immunologically competent cells with tumor-specific antigens expressed at the cell surface (Old, 1981). Such antigens are usually introduced or generated by the oncogenic agent – viral or chemical – or by mutations, probably resulting from genetic instability of the tumor cells (Coulie et al., 1995), or because transplantable tumor cells arise from antigenically different hosts (Van Pel et al., 1988; Boon et al., 1989). In humans, however, it has proved much more difficult to define tumor-specific antigens, and immunotherapy has to date enjoyed only limited success. For this reason, most of the antigentic targets against which therapeutic endeavors have been directed have been lineage specific rather than tumor specific – a compromise that not only carries the attendant risk of toxicity to normal cells, but reduces the fraction of the administered agent available to destroy tumor cells. More recently, attempts have been made to induce immune responses against undefined tumor antigens, based on the observation that tumors are frequently infiltrated by lymphocytes, and that such lymphocytes may be demonstrated, in at least some cases, to react specifically with tumor cells. The therapeutic use of tumor-infiltrating lymphocytes is described in Chapter 7.

In recent years, the demonstration of a large number of abnormal, tumor-specific proteins (or, in some cases, normal proteins that are aberrantly expressed in specific neoplastic cells), generated as a consequence of the genetic lesions in tumor cells, as well as the demonstration of viral sequences in a number of human cancers have provided specific targets that can be utilized therapeutically (Gutierrez et al., 1996; Judde et al., 1996). Although the majority of the abnormal proteins relevant to neoplasia are not cell surface proteins, peptides derived from genetically altered molecules (e.g., fusion proteins) and viral proteins may be expressed at the cell surface in the context of human leucocyte antigens and are therefore capable, at least theoretically, of exciting an immune response (Klein and Klein, 1964). This new information, coupled to a much deeper knowledge of the process whereby immunocompetent cells (usually cytotoxic T lymphocytes) are activated, has led to a rekindling in the interest in immunotherapy, but for the most part – even when, for example, a hybrid protein resulting from fusion as a result of deletion or interchromosomal translocation has been identified – it has been difficult to determine whether tumor-specific peptides are expressed at the cell surface, and if so, whether they are capable of being recognized by T cells. However, immunotherapy is only one of many therapeutic approaches that can be targeted to these recently defined tumor-specific molecules. Whereas immunological approaches represent an attempt to exploit the unique or 'foreign' nature of tumor-specific proteins, nonimmunological targeting falls into two categories: approaches that, like immunotherapy, simply exploit the uniqueness of the molecular abnormalities of tumor cells, and those that depend upon a knowledge of the derangements of biochemical pathways brought about by oncogenic molecular changes.

The pathogenetic lesions in tumor cells result in inappropriate cell proliferation, increased cell lifespan, or defective differentiation. In effect, all of these lesions ultimately inhibit the exit of a given cell type from a particular differentiation compartment, and thus result in the abnormal accumulation of one or more stages in the cellular differentiation sequence. In some cases, the cell type that is accumulated and manifested as a malignant disease may vary in different phases of the disease. For example, in chronic myeloid leukemia, the predominant cell type that accumulates is the mature polymophonuclear leucocyte, but when this disease enters an accelerated phase, or blast crisis, there is progressive accumulation of immature blast cells (Clarkson and Strife, 1993) resulting from a differentiation block caused by the development of an additional genetic lesion in one of the precursor cells of the neoplastic clone (Marasca et al., 1994; Rovira et al., 1995). It is important to recognize that, as in the case of chronic myeloid leukemia, the cell type that is manifested as a neoplasm is not necessarily the only differentiation stage of the neoplastic clone, for tumor-specific therapy is only likely to be successful if directed at the 'stem cell compartment,' i.e., the proliferating cell population of the malignant clone.

Genetic lesions that are associated with cancer occur in the pathways that govern cell proliferation, differentiation, and viability. These three pathways are, at times, intimately interdigitated and tightly regulated. Thus, terminal differentiation is associated with the cessation of proliferation and sometimes with programmed cell death, or apoptosis (e.g., in cells that are continuously replaced, such as those at an epithelial surface). In the immune system, lymphocytes with reactivities against self-antigens undergo apoptosis, while the selection of immunologically reactive lymphocytes with the highest affinity for antigen also entails the apoptotic destruction of cells with lower antigen affinity. Similarly, cells in which errors occur during proliferation or differentiation are detected at cell cycle or differentiation checkpoints and, unless repair is possible, are directed into a programmed cell death pathway.

Since proliferation and differentiation are ultimately regulated by the micro-environment of the cell (Klinken, Alexander and Adams, 1988; Borzillo, Ashmun and Sherr, 1990) – note, for example, the requirements of differentiating hematopoietic stem cells for a plethora of 'colony-stimulating factors' and the broad range of growth factors and growth inhibitory factors that regulate the proliferation of all cells – cells must contain molecules (cell surface or cytoplasmic receptors) capable of recognizing the presence of external factors that control their growth, differentiation, and viability. The migration of a proliferating or differentiating cell into an alien environment, i.e., one lacking growth or viability factors able to bind to its surface receptors, will generally result in it being forced to undergo apoptosis. Tumor cells are, doubtless, equally dependent for their proliferation and survival upon such external factors (one of the more obvious examples being hormone-dependent tumors), at least during the early stages of their pathogenesis, such that they can only survive in a limited range of microenvironments. Tumor progression can be considered to be the development of an increasing ability of tumor cells to proliferate (and to survive) in microenvironments that are not normally conducive to their growth, i.e., to lose their dependence upon the presence of external factors. Thus, successful metastasis requires not only an ability to migrate through basement membranes, but also the ability to survive in environments normally hostile to the cell type in question.

Pathways to neoplasia

Autonomous growth is a consequence of genetic changes anywhere along the several pathways that extend from the micro-environmental signal itself (which could be aberrantly provided by the tumor cell), through the signal receptors and signal-transducing molecules (Kuamble et al., 1992; Golub et al., 1994), to genes that regulate the expression of the proteins necessary for DNA replication and cell division, i.e., transcription factors (Figure 2.1). Specific examples are provided in Tables 2.1 to 2.3 (see pp. 18 and 19). Because of the numerous checks and balances in these central pathways that are involved in all cellular interactions and functions, a single genetic lesion is insufficient to cause neoplasia. If successive oncogenic genetic lesions accumulate in a cell clone, they will result in a stepwise progression, each presumably associated with sufficient clonal expansion for the likelihood of

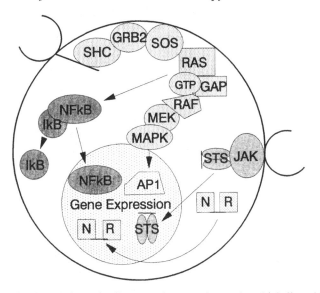

Fig. 2.1. Schematic diagram of two pathways in which ligand binding to a surface receptor triggers a cascade of events resulting in altered gene transcription. Several signal transduction pathways are shown. The Ras pathway involves a receptor tyrosine kinase and proceeds via a series of steps to mitogen-activated protein kinases (MAPK). SH2- and SH3-containing proteins, Shc and Grb2, couple the activated receptor to Ras: SOS = son of sevenless (a drosophila gene) homolog; GAP = GTPase-activating protein; MEK = MAP kinase kinase. Recent work has demonstrated that Ras can influence other signaling pathways and does not operate solely through the Raf/MAPK pathway. One such pathway is that involving the transcription factor NFkB. Others involve genes not shown here, including *Rac1* and *RhoA* which are important for actin cytoskeletal organization. In the JAK–STAT (Jak-STS) pathway, the STAT proteins are components of a DNA-binding protein complex formed predominantly in response to cytokines binding to their receptors. The STAT are translocated to the nucleus where they activate their target genes. Nuclear receptors – a large family which includes steroid hormone and retinoic acid receptors – are also shown. When ligand binds to cytoplasmic receptor these protein complexes are translocated to the nucleus, where they bind to their cognate DNA sequences.

a beneficial (to the potential tumor cell) mutation to arise (Figure 2.2). Eventually, a point is reached at which the clone has acquired sufficient autonomy for the accumulated cells to be expressed as a cancer (Klein and Klein, 1985; Vogelstein and Kinzler, 1993). The latter may initially be limited to a single microenvironment, but may continue to accumulate genetic lesions which may activate cellular pathways associated with metastasis, including the ability to survive in a broader range of microenvironments.

In most neoplasms, genetic lesions in both oncogenes, i.e., growth-promoting genes, and growth-suppressor genes, i.e., genes with a role in cell

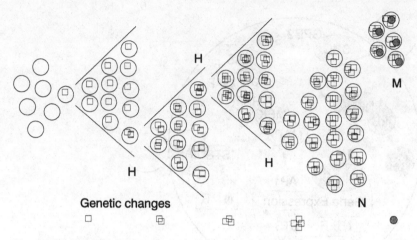

Fig. 2.2. Schematic diagram depicting the stepwise accumulation of genetic defects (five are shown here) leading, via hyperplasia, to neoplasia and tumor progression. Each genetic abnormality either provides the cell clone that contains it with a progressive growth advantage, or predisposes to the occurrence of additional genetic changes. In either event, the selection of advantageous mutations must involve clonal expansion. In this figure, only genetic changes advantageous to pathogenesis or progression are shown – many may have a deleterious effect, or have no growth- or differentiation-related consequences. H = hyperplasia, N = neoplasia, M = metastasis.

cycle checkpoints (Figure 2.3), are present. In other words, the guardians of legitimate proliferation or differentiation, which prevent the replication of damaged or imperfectly differentiated cells, must themselves be inactivated (either at the level of detection of the abnormality, or in the apoptosis pathway that is linked to the checkpoints) if the consequences of oncogene overactivity are to be expressed as neoplasia. Lymphocytes, for example, require at least two signals to induce proliferation. One signal in the absence of the other will activate a checkpoint and induce apoptosis (Evans et al., 1994). Similarly, cells with aberrantly expressed growth-promoting genes (i.e., expressed in the absence of appropriate signals from the cell surface) consequent upon genetic change will trigger diversion to an apoptotic pathway (Figure 2.4; Chiarugi et al., 1994). Perhaps not surprisingly, therefore, mutations or deletions of inhibitory genes involved in the G1 checkpoint, including *p53*, *p15/p16*, *p19*, and *CdK4*, are frequently observed in cancer. Inherited mutations of these genes have also been described in families or individuals with cancer predispositions: *p16* mutations are associated with melanoma and pancreatic cancer, *Rb* mutations with retinoblastoma and osteogenic sarcoma, and *p53* mutations with sarcomas, leukemias, brain tumors, and early onset breast cancer (the Li–Fraumeni syndrome).

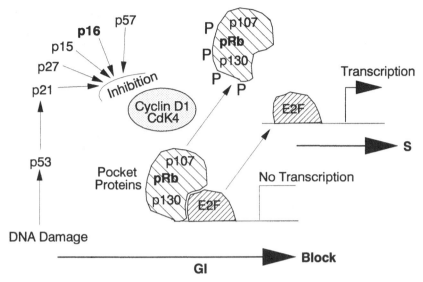

Fig. 2.3. Schematic diagram depicting the cell cycle G1 checkpoint. Cyclin D/CdK4 or Cyclin D/CdK6 complexes are formed when external events (growth factor binding to receptors) induce their synthesis. This complex phosphorylates one of the so-called pocket proteins (the Rb protein being the most critical member), which, when hypophosphorylated, prevent the transcription factor, E2F (in fact a family of at least five proteins which form heterodimers with another family of proteins known as DP), from transactivating its target genes. Phosphorylated Rb releases E2F, which initiates transcription. At least some of the target genes of E2F are involved in progression through the cell cycle and DNA synthesis. However, in some circumstances, E2F can induce apoptosis. This may account for the ability of at least one member of the E2F family, E2F-1, to function both as an oncogene and a tumor suppressor gene. G1 arrest results when this mechanism is disrupted, e.g., through ligand binding (e.g., tumor growth factor-β induces the cyclin kinase inhibitor, p27), or mutation of the inhibitors of cyclin D-kinase (e.g., p16), the kinase complex itself, or a pocket protein, particularly Rb. DNA damage, e.g., through radiation or exposure to alkylating agents, can also cause G1 arrest, via p53 expression. p53 induces the cyclin kinase inhibitor, p21. During S phase, E2F function is inhibited by a mechanism involving binding to cyclin A-kinase, which releases E2F from DNA. Failure of this mechanism results in G2 arrest and may, as when G1 arrest occurs, lead to apoptosis.

In similar fashion, neoplastic cells, or potential neoplastic cells that undergo differentiation (i.e., a neoplasm in which the primary genetic aberration occurs in an immature cell but the neoplasm is expressed as a more mature cell type) must pass differentiation checkpoints in which the integrity of an essential component of differentiation (e.g., expression of a functional immunoglobulin molecule in a B lymphocyte) is assessed before the cell is allowed to replicate. Once again, cells which fail to pass muster are diverted to a pathway leading to apoptosis (Liebermann and Hoffman, 1994). The cell cycle checkpoints

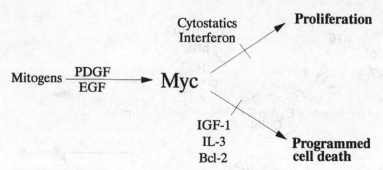

Fig. 2.4. Diagrammatic depiction of alternative consequences of *Myc* expression. Overexpression of *Myc* in the absence of growth factors such as platelet-derived growth factor (PDGF) or epidermal growth factor (EGF) leads to apoptosis rather than cell proliferation. This can be prevented by exposure of cells to insulin-like growth factor-1 (IGF-1), interleukin-3 (IL-3) or by Bcl-2, which inhibit apoptosis.

are exquisitely tuned and highly efficient. Even so, since billions of cells undergo cell division every day in each of us, even random genetic errors that may occur only once in several billion cell divisions are certain to occur frequently, particularly at a human population level (Hartwell and Kastan, 1994). Whether or not they are manifested as neoplasia depends upon whether additional genetic changes are already present, or develop in the cell.

Recently, an additional difference between many tumor cells and normal somatic cells, which appears to be separable from proliferation and differentiation pathways, was described. This is the expression of the enzyme telomerase (Kim et al., 1994), which is detectable in most, but not all, malignant tumors. Telomerase is responsible for adding repeat sequences to the terminal region of chromosomal DNA. Under normal circumstances, the number of repeat sequences is diminished each time a cell replicates. Since the presence of a minimal number of such repeats is essential to normal chromosomal replication, the number of proliferation cycles that a cell can pass through is limited in the absence of telomerase. In germ cells, telomerase is able to add additional repeat sequences to terminal DNA, in effect making such cells immortal. How tumor cells are able to express telomerase, in contradistinction to their normal counterpart cells, is unknown, but this enzyme, although not truly tumor specific, also represents a potential therapeutic target (Feng et al., 1995).

In order to grow beyond a certain size, tumors must be able to stimulate the growth of new blood vessels to provide the necessary oxygen and nutrients (Bikfalvi, 1995; Folkman, 1995a, 1995b); while to metastasize to other tissues or organs, tumor cells must also develop the ability to cross basement membranes (in order to enter and leave the bloodstream or lymphatic channels). Although at first sight these requirements appear to be grossly aberrant, migration and the stimulation of angiogenesis are in fact essential components of embryogenesis, while some normal cells retain the ability to migrate through normal tissues (e.g., cells of the immune system) or to stimulate the growth of new lymphatic and blood vessels (e.g., muscle undergoing hypertrophy and regenerating organs or tissues). Angiogenesis induction and migration through basement membranes may be normal attributes of some cell types, or may require lesions in relatively few genes, since the expression of the multiple proteins involved is likely to be regulated by a small number of (or even a single) transcription factors – master genes that have multiple target genes. The genes involved with angiogenesis and metastasis, which are abnormally expressed by cancer cells, also represent legitimate therapeutic targets (Baillie, Winslet and Bradley, 1995; Folkman, 1995c; Hawkins, 1995; Martiny-Baron and Marme, 1995; Rak, St Croix and Kerbel, 1995; Teicher, 1995).

Tumorigenesis involves a process of selection: each step towards automony can be taken only by the single cell that developed the genetic change that gave it a survival advantage (see Figure 2.2). There can be little doubt, however, that the chance of such a genetic change developing is increased by the presence of the previous genetic changes, some of which may cause genetic instability (e.g., lesions in genes involved in the detection of DNA damage or repair) (Nowell, 1976; Fishel and Kolodner, 1995; Radman et al., 1995).

Types of genetic lesions in cancer cells

The genetic lesions that lead to cancer include chromosomal translocations, intergenic or intragenic deletions, point mutations or partial or complete gene amplifications. Altered expression of proto-oncogenes, i.e., genes that directly promote cell growth, are dominant; only one of the two cellular alleles need be inappropriately expressed for the cell to be given a 'go' signal for proliferation (Bishop, 1991). In constrast, in the case of tumor suppressor genes, or genes that promote apoptosis, both alleles must normally be inactivated, either by deletion or mutation, in order for there to be a functional result (Harris, 1992). In some situations, however, reduced gene dosage caused by inactivation by one of the alleles of a tumor suppressor gene (e.g. *p53*) may have functional consequences.

The growth-promoting pathway extends from the cell surface (receptors) to the nucleus (transcription factors) and connects the external microenviron-

Table 2.1. *Genetic abnormalities involving receptors*

Malignancy	Ligand/receptor	Type of lesion
Glioblastoma, breast	PDGF receptor	Overexpression
Squamous carcinomas	EGF receptor	Overexpression
Breast, ovary, non-small cell lung cancer	Her2/neu	Overexpression
Anaplastic large cell lymphoma	Alk	Fusion with nucleophosmin
Chronic myeloid leukemia	Abl	Fusion with bcr
Chronic myeloid leukemia	PDGF receptor	Fusion with Tel
Thyroid carcinoma	Trk	Fusion with Tpr
Gastric carcinoma	Met	Fusion with Tpr
Neuroblastoma	Neu	Point mutations
Leukemia	Neu	Point mutations

Table 2.2. *Genetic abnormalities involving signal transduction pathway genes*

Malignancy	Gene	Type of lesion
Pancreatic cancer (90–95%)	*Ki-Ras*	Point mutation
Colon adenocarcinoma (20–45%)	*Ki-Ras* and *N-Ras*	Point mutation
Thyroid carcinoma (40–65%)	*Ki-Ras*, *Ha-ras* and *N-ras*	Point mutation
Lung carcinoma (7–25%)	*Ki-Ras*	Point mutation

ment of the cell to the cell proliferation cycle. Genetic lesions in receptor molecules (cell surface or cytoplasmic) involved in growth stimulation (Table 2.1) usually result in activation of the receptor protein – i.e., the effect is similar to that which would occur in the continuous presence of ligand. Sometimes the ligand-binding portion of the receptor may be lost, the cytoplasmic portion being, as a consequence, constitutively activated (e.g., with respect to a kinase function) such that the entire signal transduction pathway is activated (Cheatham et al., 1993; Morris et al., 1994). In other cases, proteins on the signal transduction pathway itself may be constitutively activated as a result of mutations, by far the most common of these in proteins of the *ras* gene family (Table 2.2). Mutations in the *Nf-1* gene, a protein with GTPase-activating activity, have been associated with a predisposition to the development of tumors, presumably resulting from an inability to convert Ras-associated GTP to GDP, thus maintaining *ras* in its active, i.e., signal-transmitting, form (Hall, 1992; Satoh and Kaziro, 1992), even in the absence of a signal. The terminus of the signal transduction pathway (transcription factors) is also a frequent target for the genetic changes that give rise to cancer (Table 2.3).

Table 2.3. *Genetic abnormalities involving transcription factors*

Malignancy	Gene	Chromosome(s)	Type of lesion
Lymphomas (B and T)	*Myc*	8;14,8;22,2;8	Enhancer juxtaposition
Lymphomas	*Tcl3/Hox11*	10;14	Enhancer juxtaposition
ALL (precursor B)	*Pbx-E2A*	1;19	Chimeric gene
ALL (precursor T)	*Scl/Tal-1*	1;14 1 interstitial deletion	Enhancer or Sil juxtaposition
Acute promyelocytic leukemia	*Rarα;Pml*	15;17	Chimeric gene
Acute myeloid leukemia	*Aml1-Eto*	8;21	Chimeric gene
Acute myeloid leukemia	*All1-Af9*	9;11	Chimeric gene
Many cancers	*p53*	17	Deletion or point mutation

Overexpression, or inappropriate expression, of a proto-oncogene is caused either by gene amplification or by alteration in the regulatory region of the gene, resulting in increased or inappropriate transcription. Mutations that inactivate suppressor regions in or near gene promoters may be sufficient to result in abnormal expression, but the presence of gross structural changes in chromosomes with resultant juxtaposition of two genes normally separated in the genome is also frequently observed. The structural consequences that lead to increased transcription include juxtaposition of the regulatory region (but not the promoter) of one gene to the promoter of another (frequently with deletion or mutation of the regulatory elements of the latter), resulting in the deregulation of the gene (Magrath, 1990). This is a common theme in lymphoid neoplasia, in which chromosomal translocations or intragenic deletions result in the juxtaposition of proto-oncogenes to the regulatory regions of antigen receptor genes (either immunoglobulin or T cell antigen receptor genes) such that the proto-oncogenes (which may or may not normally be expressed in the cell type in which the genetic change occurs) are expressed in situations in which the antigen receptor gene would normally be expressed (Figure 2.5a). This, in essence, results in constitutive expression of the proto-oncogene, since antigen receptor genes are, in general, expressed continuously in lymphocytes. Examples of this type of translocation include those in which the *c-myc* gene, normally resident on chromosome 8, band q24, is juxtaposed to immunoglobulin or Tα regulatory sequences (Gutierrez, Bhatia and Barriga, 1992). In other translocations, a proto-oncogene may be juxtaposed, in frame, to the promoter of another gene. The latter need only

(a)

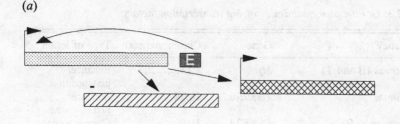

(b)

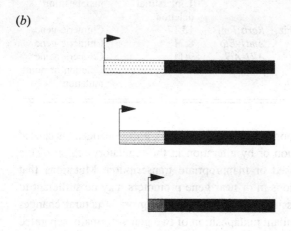

(c)

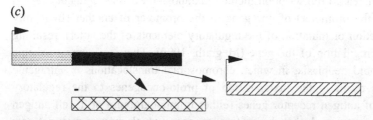

Fig. 2.5. Diagrammatic depiction of several types of translocation involving transcription factors. (*a*) Juxtaposition of a transcription factor to enhancer elements. This type of translocation is common in lymphomas such as Burkitt's lymphoma, in which *c-myc* is juxtaposed to immunoglobulin enhancer elements, and some T cell leukemias, in which *c-myc* is juxtaposed to T cell receptor enhancer elements. (*b*) Promiscuous use of alternative promoters (often as many as 12) in the formation of a chimeric transcription factor. This occurs in leukemias and lymphomas, for example genes such as *ALL-1* (from chromosome 11q23) and *Bcl-6* (on chromosome 3q). (*c*) Formation of chimeric transcription factors, as is common in several solid tumors, and acute leukemias (see text). In leukemias, the core binding transcription factor, which binds to enhancer elements in a number of genes relevant to hemopoiesis, is particularly frequently involved (see Okuda et al., 1996).

be a gene that is expressed in the normal counterpart cells of the neoplasm, and the same end result may be achieved by juxtaposition to one of several alternative promoters (sometimes known as 'promiscuous translocation'), as occurs in translocations involving the *bcl-6* gene normally situated on chromosome 3 band q27 (Deweindt et al., 1993; Ye et al., 1993), or the *ALL-1* gene situated on chromosome 11q23 (Figure 2.5b).

In a third type of translocation, not only the promoter, but a significant part of one gene may be fused to another, creating a chimeric protein (Figure 2.5c; Rabbits, 1991; Golub et al., 1994). Once again, this is a common theme in hematopoietic neoplasia, the gene pairs involved in the fusion most often being transcription factors, or proteins that modulate the ability of transcription factors to regulate the expression of other genes. In some cases the genetic abnormalities result in increased transcription of growth-promoting genes', in others, they cause reduction of the expression of growth-suppressor genes (Figure 2.6). This concept, however, may be an oversimplification since many of these transcription factors may affect many genes, in some cases suppressing, in others increasing, transcription. One of the partners in the fusion protein is normally expressed in the normal counterpart cell of the neoplasm, while the other is not. Thus, the functional consequences of such translocations include inappropriate or aberrant expression of a transactivating function (specified by the DNA-binding region which is aberrantly expressed in the chimeric protein), altered specificity for target genes (brought about, for example, by modification of the DNA-binding region), or inhibition of a transactivating (or repressor) function. The regulation of gene expression always entails the participation of many proteins and the formation of homodimers or heterodimers. Thus, inhibition may be brought about by overexpression of an inhibitory protein aberrantly expressed as a chimeric protein, or the creation of a new inhibitory molecule from expression of a modified transcription factor still capable of dimerization, but now exerting an inhibitory effect on the normal protein (a dominant negative effect).

Excellent examples of genetic lesions in transcription factors are provided by the hematopoietic malignancies. The components of the heterodimeric core-binding factor (CBF), which binds to an enhancer element present in a number of genes involved in hematopoiesis, including the T cell antigen receptor, are frequent targets of translocations resulting in fusion genes in acute myeloid and acute lymphoid leukemias. In the 8;21 translocation AML-1 (CBFα) forms a fusion gene with a putative zinc-finger transcription factor, ETO. AML-1 forms several alternative fusion genes in the 3;21 translocation that occurs occasionally in myelodysplasia and in blast transformation of chronic myeloid leukemia, and a chimeric transcription factor with the *TEL*

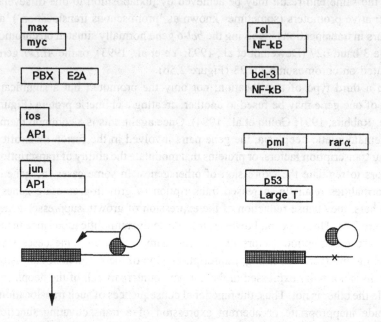

Fig. 2.6. Combinatorial associations of various members of regulatory proteins able to influence transcription of genes containing their cognate response elements. myc:max heterodimers transactivate genes containing E-box response elements. The PBX-E2A chimeric gene created by the 1;19 chromosomal translocation which occurs in a subset of precursor B cell acute lymphoblastic leukemia cells deregulates transcription in genes containing E2F sites. Both Fos and Jun proteins, which form a heterodimer able to bind to AP1 sites, are oncogenic when overexpressed. Some combinatorial associations are dominant negative. Thus the association of IkB with NF-kB prevents translation of the latter transcription factor to the nucleus. Rel, a protein related to the DNA-binding and dimerization domains of NF-kB, can prevent IkB's inhibitory effects. Sequestration of p53 by large T antigen results in prevention of p53 growth inhibitory function (other viral genes, *E6* and *E1a*, cause similar loss of p53 function by causing its degradation).

gene, a member of the *ETS* family, in approximately 25% of cases of acute lymphoblastic leukemia. In the inversion of chromosome 16 (in essence, an intrachromosomal translocation between 16q22 and 16p13), which occurs particularly in M4 leukemia associated with eosinophilia, CBFβ forms a fusion gene with a smooth muscle myosin heavy chain, MYH11. The chimeric protein is still able to dimerize with CBFα via the CBFβ component, but myosin multimers are now brought into the vicinity of the complex of enzymes

(*a*)

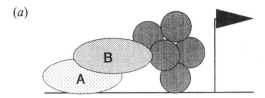

(*b*)

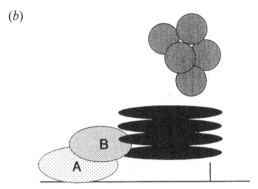

Fig. 2.7. Inhibition of transcription by the CBFβ-MYH11 chimeric protein created by the inv(16) seen in acute myelomonocytic leukemia. (*a*) Transcription normally occurs when the AML-1 (CBFα)–CBFβ complex binds to an enhancer element in the gene. (*b*) Hypothetical depiction of interference in the formation of the transcriptional complex by the fusion protein involving CBFβ and a myosin heavy chain.

necessary for transcription, and probably physically interferes with the final assembly of the transcriptional complex on the promoter (Figure 2.7).

It is clear from the above discussion that in most cases, the development of therapeutic approaches directed at transformation-specific targets requires a reasonably detailed knowledge of the biochemical consequences of the genetic changes present in tumor cells. Such knowledge, however, should permit the development of potentially exquisite tumor cell specificity since the targets are not present in normal cells. Moreover, since the targets are essential to the continued existence of the neoplastic cell (genetic changes associated with tumor progression do not fall into this category), it should, theoretically, prove difficult for resistance to the therapeutic approach to develop.

Transformation-specific therapeutic approaches

Transformation-specific therapeutic approaches can be divided into those in which the intent is to reverse the consequence of a particular genetic change (e.g., downregulation or inhibition of the function of an overexpressed gene; replacement of a missing function), and those in which the genetic lesion is simply used as a trigger to initiate the expression of a 'suicide gene' that will cause cell death – either by directly inducing apoptosis (Cirielli et al., 1995; Santoso et al., 1995) or by activating a therapeutic agent, such as a prodrug, delivered separately to the patient (Table 2.4). For present purposes, these two quite different approaches are referred to as *reversion therapy*, in which the functional consequences of one or more of the genetic lesions present in a tumor are reversed, and *assisted suicide*, in which the tumor-specific lesions are used to activate a separate therapeutic system which causes cell death (Gutierrez et al., 1996). Both approaches are associated with innate difficulties which, in some cases, are not surmountable by presently available technology. Particularly problematic, when therapy is dependent upon a vectored gene, is the need for the gene to reach every tumor cell capable of proliferating (except when there is a significant 'bystander' effect – see below).

The degree of tumor specificity achieved with therapy directed to transformation-specific targets will depend upon the details of the approach used. Reversion therapy, for example, if directed towards proteins that are simply overexpressed in tumor cells, may not be without toxicity in some normal cells, but may still produce a sufficient differential toxicity to make it an acceptable therapeutic approach, e.g., agents such as farnesyl transferase inhibitors directed against *ras* genes, or tyrosine kinase inhibitors (Murakami et al., 1988; Yuan, Jakes and Elliot, 1990; Dvir et al., 1991; Gibbs, Oliff and Kohl, 1994). This is, of course, the basis for conventional chemotherapeutic and radiotherapeutic agents, but at least some targeted agents could prove to have a higher therapeutic index than conventional agents. In the case of assisted suicide, the activated therapeutic system may itself be nonspecific (Huber et al., 1993), e.g., a drug or toxin, but tumor specificity is predicated upon release within tumor cells. If, however, either the activating or activated agent is capable of egression from the tumor cell, some loss of specificity will take place. This bystander effect, which refers to the death of cells in the vicinity of the successfully targeted cells, may have advantages where the targeting vehicle reaches only a fraction of the tumor cells, since a high proportion of the cells immediately adjacent to those that are successfully targeted will be tumor cells. However, the bystander effect could also, depending upon its magnitude, dilute the tumor specificity of the system either

Table 2.4. *A classification of transformation-dependent targeted therapy*

A. Reversion therapy
Inhibition therapy
1. Sequence-specific therapy.
   e.g., antisense, ribozyme, triplex therapy
2. Aberrant protein-specific therapy
   e.g., drugs developed via peptide inhibition, protein-dependent inhibition via transduced constructs
Gene replacement therapy
e.g., replacement of a deleted or mutated tumor suppressor gene, or of certain mutated
oncogenes (*Ras*)
B. Assisted suicide
1. Tumor-specific activation of a suicide gene
   e.g., virus-directed enzyme/prodrug/therapy; lytic system, EBV dependent (LysED)
   therapy

by causing the death of adjacent normal cells (which could be of major
significance in some circumstances, such as one in which multiple metastases
are scattered throughout an organ sensitive to the toxic effects of the activated
agent), or, via entry into the bloodstream, by causing systemic toxicity. Such
toxicity may still prove to be less than that presently encountered with conventional cancer treatments. Assisted suicide systems can be rendered more highly
tumor specific by creating an effector system that is also tumor cell specific
or lineage specific such that there are two levels of tumor cell specificity –
one at the level of the activating agent, and the second at the level of the
effector system (Gutierrez et al., 1996). This is discussed further below.

Reversion therapy

Reversion therapy falls into two categories: inhibition of an overexpressed
gene product (i.e., of an oncogene) or replacement of a missing function (i.e.,
of the product of a tumor suppressor gene). Inhibitory therapy may be directed
at the oncogene itself or its transcript, in which case it will normally be
sequence specific. Here, inhibition is achieved through targeting tumor-
specific stretches of nucleotides with RNA or DNA (McManaway et al.,
1990; see Chapter 8). Alternatively, inhibitory therapy may be directed at the
oncogene product.

Sequence-specific therapy

The objective of sequence-specific therapy is to inhibit the production of a protein that is essential to the pathogenesis of the tumor (generally a growth-promoting gene, such as *myc*) only in tumor cells, and not in normal cells. The therapeutic agent is the complementary nucleotide sequence to an oncogene, or to a part of the oncogene. It is delivered to the tumor cells either as an exogenous oligonucleotide or by means of a viral vector constructed to deliver an antisense RNA molecule. Disadvantages to the use of exogenous oligonucleotides are that degradation may be rapid in either serum or the cell, and penetration into cells may be inadequate or require very high concentrations of the oligonucleotide. Degradation can be minimized by chemical modifications such as methylation or the addition of thiol groups (Stein, 1992; Stein and Cohen, 1988), or by delivery in a protective system such as a liposome. An additional disadvantage, however, is that the oligonucleotide is distributed throughout the body, into all normal cells. While tumor specificity of the therapeutic molecule may minimize normal tissue toxicity, greatest efficiency and safety would result from conferring some degree of tumor specificity onto the delivery of the agent. One approach to this problem is to use liposomal delivery (Akhtar et al., 1991), and to confer some tissue or cellular specificity onto the liposome, for example by incorporating a monoclonal antibody into it (Wang and Huang, 1987). The success of such approaches remains to be demonstrated. Using a vector to deliver the sequence-specific therapeutic molecule avoids the problem of enzymatic degradation, and has additional possibilities for tumor specificity – specificity for tumor cells can be engineered into the surface proteins of a viral vector, or the therapeutic molecule could be made dependent upon a gene expressed only in the tumor cell (Figure 2.8). In addition, once the vector has entered the cell, use of appropriate promoters can ensure that high levels of antisense or triplex molecules are delivered.

Sequence-specific inhibition of the gene in question can be accomplished either by using a nucleotide sequence that will form a region of triplex DNA with the gene in question or its regulatory sequence, or through the use of antisense (or ribozyme) molecules to inhibit the translation of mRNA. Such approaches could be used to inhibit the expression of an unmodified, inappropriately or overexpressed growth-promoting gene, including tumor-specific chimeric genes, or a gene that endows a prolonged lifespan on the cell, for example, *bcl-2* (Perrouault et al., 1990; Cheng et al., 1992; Yang, Cedergren and Nada-Ginard, 1994; Cai, Mukhopadhyay and Roth, 1995). At the present time, the inhibition of a gene in vivo by the formation of a triplex molecule is extremely difficult to accomplish for a variety of technical reasons (see

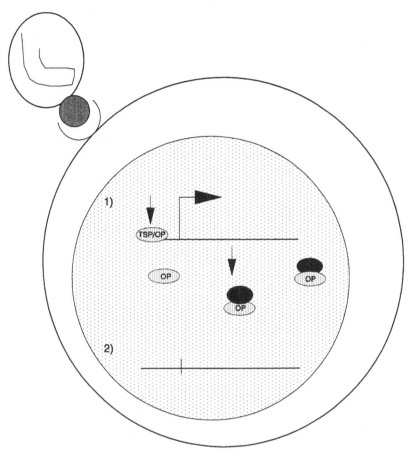

Fig. 2.8. Levels at which specificity could be introduced in a vectored system of gene targeting. Firstly, the vector itself (liposome or virus) could be rendered specific for a receptor expressed only on a limited fraction of cells. Secondly, expression of the therapeutic (inhibitory) protein could be regulated either by a tumor-specific protein (TSP) e.g. alpha-fetoprotein (i.e., the promoter that drives the inhibitory protein incorporates a regulatory element used by alpha-fetoprotein, which is only expressed in the tumor cells), or even by the oncoprotein (oncogene or dominant negative antioncogene) itself when this is a transcription factor. (1) When the oncoprotein (OP) is present, transcription of the inhibitory protein or peptide occurs. (2) When the oncoprotein is absent, as is the case in normal cells, transcription of the inhibitory protein does not occur. Once the inhibitory protein is in excess, transcription will no longer be driven since no oncoprotein will be available. This would allow the inhibitory effect to be overcome with time, but would not be of importance if inhibition of the tumor-specific molecule led to apoptosis (e.g., inhibition of a mutated *p53* gene). Neither of these two levels is necessarily absolutely tumor specific, but together they confer a high degree of specificity. In addition, the third degree of specificity is built into the inhibitory protein/peptide itself, which could be constructed such that it inhibits only the oncoprotein, where this is unique, i.e., a chimeric or mutated protein.

Chapter 8), so that most sequence-specific therapy is limited to the use of antisense or ribozyme molecules (Szczylik et al., 1991; Gewirtz, 1993; Skorski et al., 1993; Smetsers et al., 1994). Operationally, these approaches are identical, in that both, if effective, result in the inhibition of translation. Whereas antisense molecules may or may not result in destruction of the message to which they bind, ribozymes contain a sequence-specific element responsible for their specificity and a catalytic unit that destroys the RNA molecule. A variation on this theme is the use of 2γ-5γ oligoantisense chimera molecules in which an agent capable of inducing the degradation of the mRNA is coupled to the antisense molecule. Examples of tumor-specific antisense therapy which have been shown to be effective, at least in vitro, include the use of an antisense oligomer directed to the tumor-specific intron sequences that persist in *c-myc* mRNA in some Burkitt's lymphomas (McManaway et al., 1990), or to a hybrid message such as *bcr-abl* transcripts present in chronic myeloid leukemia (including blast crises) or subtypes of acute lymphoblastic leukemia (Szczylik et al., 1991; Smetsers et al., 1994).

Protein-directed inhibition

Mutated or chimeric proteins, being tumor specific, provide excellent targets for therapy. Either other proteins, or peptides as well as, in theory, a variety of other compounds (i.e., drugs) may be used to inhibit their function. The use of proteins or peptides as inhibitory molecules is particularly well suited to mutated or chimeric proteins (Szczylik et al., 1991; Skorski et al., 1993). In the context of mutated proteins, the feasibility of this approach is demonstrated by the existence of antibodies which will bind to a mutated protein but not to its normal counterpart, and by the fact that the conformational changes brought about by the mutation may alter the pattern of binding to other proteins (mutated *p53* provides an excellent example of both of these phenomena). Proteins that are not themselves abnormal but that are expressed aberrantly may also provide therapeutic targets, although in this case tumor specificity is not inherent in the protein itself, but, if desired, must be created at a different level (see below). The inhibition of such normal, but aberrantly expressed proteins at the protein level can be accomplished by a variety of methods, including by chemical compounds screened for their ability to inhibit the protein's function, by the introduction of an excess of another protein or peptide capable of binding to and inhibiting the function of the pathogenic molecule, or, in some cases, by the use of drugs. In the special case of transcription factors, an additional method can be considered: introduction of a sufficient quantity of the cognate DNA sequence to which the transcription factor normally binds into the cell ('decoy' therapy). As with antisense therapy, this approach may be attempted either through exposure of cells to oligonucleotide (necessarily double stranded), or through transduction of the cells with viral sequences, or expression vectors which will create multimeric forms of the cognate sequences. Clearly, it would be necessary to test these various approaches first in the specific systems into which they might be introduced, in vitro.

Failing more direct approaches of identifying inhibitory molecules, it would be necessary to develop a means of screening large numbers of compounds for their ability to inhibit a tumor-specific protein. The development of such assay systems may be relatively straightforward in the case of transcription factors, where the ability of compounds to inhibit the expression of a readily assayed reporter gene (e.g., luciferase) driven by a functional tumor-specific protein (or pathogenetically relevant viral protein), or to prevent the inhibition of the reporter gene, can be readily tested (Figure 2.9). Unfortunately, the screening process itself is likely to be extremely lengthy unless data exist regarding the probable structure of compounds likely to be inhibitory. An alternative, and more immediately feasible, strategy, which is not solely

(*a*)

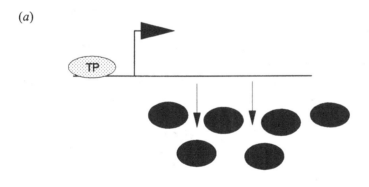

(*b*)

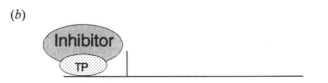

Fig. 2.9. Principle of an in-vitro assay system for the screening of molecules that inhibit a transcription factor. A reporter gene, driven by the transcription factor/protein (TP) is not synthesized in the presence of inhibitors of the transcription factor.

applicable to transcription factors, is to use other proteins or peptides as potential inhibitors (Gibbs, 1992; Amati et al., 1993; Huber, Koblan and Heimbrook, 1994). Sometimes it may be possible to introduce known inhibitory molecules into the tumor cell (e.g., max or mad, when *c-myc* is overexpressed), although such an approach is only likely to be successful when the delivery system is engineered to be tumor specific. Where a putatively normal oncoprotein is known to dimerize, the use of a modified version of the protein itself can be contemplated. For example, in the case of a transcription factor which can only bind DNA in dimeric form, inhibition may be achieved by introducing a version of the protein into the tumor cell that is unable to bind DNA, but which can still dimerize with the normal protein. This 'dominant negative' phenomenon is a theme that occurs in oncogenesis; some mutated growth-suppressor genes (e.g., *p53*) are able to bind to the unmutated protein and inhibit its function — both alleles are inactivated even though only one is mutated. Variations on this theme can be envisaged, the precise strategy adopted depending upon the nature of the genetic change in the oncoprotein or growth-suppressor gene. For example, a normal heterodimeric partner could be engineered such that it renders the dimeric complex afunctional.

Even in the case of mutant or chimeric molecules in which there are no known partner proteins, a rapid screening method could be employed to identify proteins or peptides that will bind to the aberrant protein. (The functional consequences would then need to be determined.) For example, large numbers (millions) of random peptides can be readily generated and coupled to beads or expressed by bacteriophages. Specific binding of one or more peptides to the protein of choice can then be identified by a suitable assay system (O'Neil and Hoess, 1995; Schumacher et al., 1996). Such approaches are frequently used to identify epitopes recognized by monoclonal antibodies (Luders et al., 1985).

The identification of previously unrecognized proteins which bind to mutated or chimeric oncoproteins may be achieved by standard cloning systems using cDNA libraries, or by a version of the 'two hybrid' assay (Allen et al., 1995), depicted in Figure 2.10. Subsequently it would be necessary either to develop a tumor-specific means of delivery (see below), or chemically to modify the structure of the protein, protein domain or peptide, such that it would have no effect on the normal counterparts of tumor-specific proteins. The modified molecule could be used as a drug, or its cognate DNA could be molecularly cloned into a vector (e.g., a retrovirus or adenovirus) suitable for transduction and expression in tumor cells. Various approaches to rendering delivery specific for tumor cells exist, including rendering the vector tumor or lineage specific, or even requiring the presence of the same oncogene for expression of the therapeutic agent (see Figure 2.8).

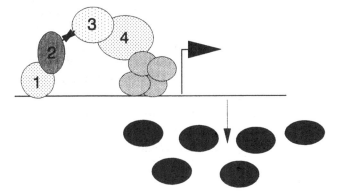

Fig. 2.10. Principle of the two hybrid system for rapid screening of proteins that bind to other proteins. The target protein (2) is coupled to the DNA-binding region (1) of a transcription factor (e.g., yeast Gal4), and transfected into a suitable cell type (usually a yeast cell). Next, a cDNA library is constructed (3) and inserted in the vector immediately upstream of the transactivating region of the transcription factor (4). When the cDNA library is transfected into yeast cells containing the target protein/ transcription factor hybrid, transactivation of the gene – in this case *gal4* – will occur only if the library contains a protein encoded in (3) that is able to bind to the target protein (2). The reporter gene is chosen for its readily measurable product, in the case of *gal4*, galactose.

Replacement therapy

Replacement therapy is gene therapy in the purest sense, i.e., replacement of a missing function caused by genetic deletion or point mutation. Such genes will normally either be tumor suppressor genes or apoptosis-inducing genes. The feasibility of reversal of the malignant phenotype by this approach has been clearly demonstrated by replacement of mutated *p53* or *Rb* genes in a variety of tumor cell lines (Huang et al., 1988; Baket et al., 1990; Bookstein et al., 1990; Cheng et al., 1992; Cai et al., 1993; Fujiwara et al., 1994) and more recently of inhibitory proteins of cell cycle progression (e.g., *p21, p16*). As with inhibitory therapy, it would appear prudent to utilize tumor-specific or tissue-specific delivery systems for gene replacement therapy to avoid untoward effects on normal cells caused by increased gene dosage, although attempts have been made to introduce viral constructs containing the relevant replacement gene into the tumor itself or into an anatomically defined compartment containing the tumor (e.g., bladder, mouth, peritoneum), such that exposure to the vector will be limited to normal epithelium (see Chapter 4).

Assisted suicide

Any of the targeting approaches already discussed may be used to trigger a
suicide gene in tumor cells, but many of these approaches ultimately depend
upon the delivery to the tumor cell of a therapeutic modality that is not tumor
specific. The conferring of tumor specificity on drugs or prodrugs by coupling
them to targeting molecules such as triplex or antisense molecules or, less
specifically, monoclonal antibodies or receptor ligands, is closely related to
the assisted suicide approach, but, with the exception of sequence-specific
therapy directed to tumor-specific sequences (McManaway et al., 1990;
Skorski et al., 1993), does not fall within the realm of transformation-directed
therapy. In addition, assisted suicide refers to a therapeutic agent that is
activated only in a tumor cell, not one that is simply targeted to a tumor
cell. Various approaches, including the use of tumor-specific expression of
prodrug-converting enzymes (discussed in Chapter 4), apoptosis-inducing
genes, or viral genes (see below) can be envisaged.

Targeting pathogenetically relevant viral genes

Strictly speaking, viral genes that contribute to tumorigenesis cannot be considered to be genetic abnormalities. For our purposes, however, viral genes
can be considered the equivalent of aberrantly expressed cellular genes that
are capable of interacting with other cellular genes or proteins and so contributing to oncogenesis. The E6 protein of the tumorigenic human papilloma virus
strains, for example, induces rapid degradation of cellular *p53* in a subset
of cervical cancers (Bornstein, Rahat and Abramovici, 1995), which is the
equivalent of a deletion or mutation in *p53*. Where viral proteins relevant to
oncogenesis have been identified, approaches to genetic intervention can be
devised. Thus, inhibition of E6 should result in the normal expression and
function of *p53* in such cells. Similarly, inhibition of E7, which binds and
inhibits the retinoblastoma protein, Rb, should permit normal Rb function.
As predicted, inhibition of both E6 and E7 by antisense has been shown to
result in reversion of the tumorigenic phenotype in a cervical cancer cell line
(Hu et al., 1995).

Another DNA virus that is associated with human malignancy, ranging
from lymphomas to epithelial cancers, is Epstein–Barr virus (EBV). We
have previously presented evidence that *EBNA-1* may be relevant to the
pathogenesis of EBV-associated Burkitt's lymphoma, and since this gene is
responsible for maintenance of episomal copies of the viral genome (Yates
et al., 1984), its inhibition should result in loss of EBV from tumor cells. As

long as EBV is relevant to the maintenance of the transformed phenotype, regardless of which latent genes are involved, its loss from the cell will result in reversal of the transformed state.

Even when viral genes have not been demonstrated to be relevant to pathogenesis, expressed viral genes could be used in assisted suicide therapy, for example by making them targets for antibody-directed enzyme pro-drug therapy (ADEPT) (if expressed at the cell surface) or virus-directed enzyme/prodrug therapy (VDEPT) (see Chapter 4), in which the prodrug is activated by an enzyme introduced into the tumor cells and regulated by a viral gene. We have demonstrated the feasibility of this approach by introducing a cytosine deaminase gene controlled by *EBNA-1* into EBV-containing Burkitt's lymphoma cells and demonstrating tumor-specific production of 5-fluorouracil from 5-fluorocytosine with resultant cell death (Judde et al., 1996). We have also demonstrated that a second level of tumor specificity can be introduced into the system by using a tumor-specific suicide gene rather than a drug-activating enzyme. Since induction of virus production in EBV-containing cell lines results in cell lysis, and since a single viral gene, *Zebra*, is sufficient to induce virus production, we have introduced a *Zebra* gene, under the control of *EBNA-1*, into various Burkitt's lymphoma cells. This resulted, as predicted, in cell death only in EBV-positive but not in EBV-negative cells. In this case the presence of EBV is required both to cause expression of the suicide gene and to enable the latter to cause cell destruction (Figure 2.11; Gutierrez et al., 1996).

Targeting secondary components of neoplasia

The inhibition of neoangiogenesis and tumor invasion should be possible without serious toxicity to normal cells, since neither process occurs to a significant extent in normal tissues in the adult, although both are essential components of embryogenesis. Angiogenesis is an essential component of tumor growth — one form of tumor dormancy appears to result from the suppression of angiogenesis by the production by tumor cells of inhibitors of angiogenesis such as angiostatin (Folkman, 1995a, 1995b, 1995c). Tumor cells, in common with many normal cells at the time of injury or tissue hypertrophy, nearly always produce potent angiogenic molecules. Recently, evidence that endothelial cells can produce factors that influence tumor cell growth was also provided, suggesting that tumor dependency on endothelial cells sometimes goes beyond the simple requirement of a blood supply (Folkman, 1995c). Interestingly, it has also been recently shown that the enzyme tissue inhibitor metalloproteinase-2 can inhibit invasion and metastasis as

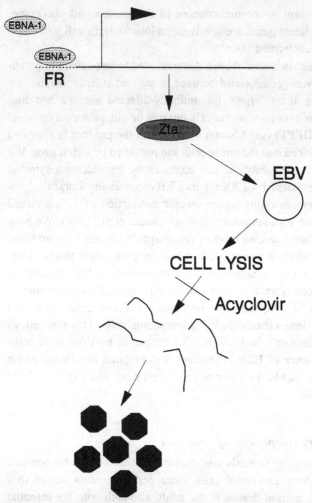

Fig. 2.11. EBV as target protein and lytic agent: two levels of specificity. The zebra protein, Zta, is necessary and sufficient for the induction of viral particles in EBV-containing cells. In this system, demonstrated to be feasible in vitro (Gutierrez et al., 1996), the Zta construct is driven by EBNA-1, an EBV latent gene expressed in all EBV-containing tumor cells. EBNA-1 is a transactivating protein which binds to the family of repeat (FR) region of the origin of plasmid replication, which can function as an enhancer. Thus, Zta is only expressed in EBV-containing cells. Since minimal numbers of normal cells contain EBV even in seropositive individuals, the system is, in effect, tumor specific with respect to Zta expression. The induction of a lytic cycle, which normally results in the production of linear viral DNA molecules and viral particles, is associated with cell lysis, such that a second level of specificity is introduced – the executor system, which causes cell death, which here is also dependent upon the presence of EBV DNA. Even when acyclovir is used to prevent viral DNA replication, cell lysis still occurs.

well as angiogenesis (Benelli et al., 1994). The use of such approaches, presumably in association with other treatment methods, could lead to a major advance over present treatment methods (Denekamp, 1984; Ingber et al., 1990; Benelli et al., 1994; Baillie, Winslet and Bradley, 1995). While neither approach should, on theoretical grounds, lead to the complete elimination of tumor, the reduction and limitation of tumor size and the prevention of further invasion provide a means of reversing the process of progression from a localized lesion to a highly invasive malignant tumor. Such therapeutic approaches may be logically used after reduction of large tumor masses by conventional means, and may subsequently be administered chronically. The production of angiogenesis inhibitors, such as angiostatin, by some tumors is one means by which tumors may remain dormant, with apoptosis exactly counterbalancing proliferation, for many years (Folkman, 1995b). Even if methods could not be found to tip the balance in favor of apoptosis, the induction of long-term tumor dormancy, if it could be accomplished, would be a rather different but entirely beneficial consequence of therapeutic expectations. While chronic administration could increase the risk of unwanted effects, and the possibility that resistance will develop, since, in the case of angiogenesis at least, the inhibitory effect is upon genetically stable cells, the development of resistance to therapy is unlikely. A small number of clinical trials of drugs that interfere with angiogenesis and metastasis are already in progress (Ingber et al., 1990; Hawkins, 1995).

Conclusion

Recent years have seen a dramatic increase in the understanding of the pathogenesis of cancer. Such knowledge brings with it the distinct possibility of developing highly tumor-specific therapeutic approaches that were inconceivable a few years ago. A number of such approaches have been shown to work in vitro, demonstrating that genetically targeted therapy is, at least in principle, feasible. A major obstacle to the success of such approaches is the difficulty of transducing a sufficiently high fraction of tumor cells; for many of the therapeutic approaches discussed, theoretically all tumor cells must be transduced. The development of more efficient methods of transducing tumor cells will be essential to the success of these approaches in patients.

One of the fascinating aspects of transformation-targeted therapy is that many of the strategies that can be envisaged are similar to those used by the tumor cell to subvert the normal cellular pathways involved in the regulation of proliferation, differentiation, and viability. Therefore, careful study of pathogenetic mechanisms is likely to provide insights into new approaches.

In addition, just as genetic lesions on several pathways – those that drive proliferation and those that regulate proliferation (cell cycle checkpoints and apoptotic pathways) – are required for the cell to become truly neoplastic, it is entirely possible that combinations of approaches will be necessary if this form of targeted therapy is to be ultimately successful. Such combinations would not only be directed towards several potential tumor targets, but may include other forms of anticancer therapy, not excluding conventional treatment and modifications in the microenvironment of the tumor cell (biological response-modifier therapy).

References

Akhtar, S., Basu, S., Wickstrom, E. et al. (1991). Interactions of antisense DNA oligonucleotide analogs with phospholipid membranes (liposomes). *Nucleic Acids Research*, **19**: 5551–9.

Allen, J. B., Walberg, M. W., Edwards, M. C. and Elledge, S. J. (1995). Finding prospective partners in the library: the two-hybrid system and phage display find a match. *Trends in Biochemical Sciences*, **20**: 511–16.

Amati, B., Brooks, M. W., Lvey, N. et al. (1993). Oncogenic activity of the c-myc protein requires dimerization with max. *Cell*, **72**: 233–45.

Baillie, C. T., Winslet, M. C. and Bradley, N. J. (1995). Tumour vasculature – a potential therapeutic target. *British Journal of Cancer*, **72**: 57–67.

Baker, S. J., Markowitz, S., Fearon, E. R. et al. (1990). Suppression of human colorectal carcinoma cell growth by wildtype p53. *Science*, **249**: 912–15.

Benelli, R., Adatia, R., Ensoli, B., Stetler-Stevenson, W. G., Santi, L. and Albini, A. (1994). Inhibition of AIDS–Kaposi's sarcoma cell induced endothelial cell invasion by TIMP-2 and a synthetic peptide from the metalloproteinase: implications for an anti-angiogenic therapy. *Oncology Research*, **6**: 251–7.

Bikfalvi, A. (1995). Significance of angiogenesis in tumour progression and metastasis. *Breast Cancer Research and Treatment*, **36**: 157–68.

Bishop, J. M. (1991). Molecular themes in oncogenesis. *Cell*, **64**: 235–48.

Boffetta, P. and Kaldor, J. M. (1994). Secondary malignancies following cancer chemotherapy. *Acta Oncologica*, **33**: 591–8.

Boice, J. D. (1988). Carcinogenesis – a synopsis of human experience with external exposure in media. *Health Physics*, **55**: 621–30.

Bookstein, R., Shew, J. Y., Chen, P. L. et al. (1990). Suppression of tumorigenicity of human prostate carcinoma cells by replacing a mutated RB gene. *Science*, **247**: 712–15.

Boon, T., Van Pel, A., De Plaen, E., Chomez, P., Lurquin, C., Szikora, J. P., Sibille, C., Mariame, B., Van den Eynde, B., Lethe, B. et al. (1989). Genes coding for T-cell-defined tum transplantation antigens: point mutations, antigenic peptides, and subgenic expression. *Cold Spring Harbor Symposium: Quantitative Biology*, **54**: 587–96.

Bornstein, J., Rahat, M. A. and Abramovici, H. (1995). Etiology of cervical cancer: current concepts. *Obstetric and Gynecological Survey*, **50**: 146–54.

Borzillo, G. V., Ashmun, R. A. and Sherr, C. J. (1990). Macrophage lineage switching of murine early pre-B lymphoid cells expressing transduced fms genes. *Molecular Cell Biology*, **10**: 2703–14.

Cai, D. W., Mukhopadhyay, T., Liu, Y. et al. (1993). Expression of the wild type p53 gene in the human lung cancer cells after retrovirus-mediated gene transfer. *Human Gene Therapy*, 4: 617–24.

Cai, D. W., Mukhopadhyay, T. and Roth, J. A. (1995). Suppression of lung cancer cell growth by ribozyme-mediated modification of p53 pre-mRNA. *Cancer Gene Therapy*, 2: 199–205.

Cheatham, B., Shoelson, S. E., Yamada, K., Goncalves, E. and Kahn, C. R. (1993). Substitution of the erbV-2 oncoprotein transmembrane domain activates the insulin receptor and modulates the action of insulin and insulin-receptor substrate 1. *Proceedings of the National Academy of Sciences of the United States of America*, 90: 7336–40.

Cheng, J., Yee, J. K., Yeargin, J. et al. (1992). Suppression of acute lymphoblastic leukemia by the human wild-type p53 gene. *Cancer Research*, 52: 222–6.

Chiarugi, V., Magnelli, L., Cinelli, M. and Basi, G. (1994). Apoptosis and the cell cycle. *Cellular and Molecular Biology Research*, 40: 603–12.

Cirielli, C., Riccioni, T., Yang, C., Pili, R., Gloe, T., Chang, J., Inyaku, K., Passaniti, A. and Capogrossi, M. C. (1995). Adenovirus-mediated gene transfer of wild-type p53 results in melanoma cell apoptosis in vitro and in vivo. *International Journal of Cancer*, 27: 673–9.

Clarkson, B. and Strife, A. (1993). Linkage of proliferative and maturational abnormalities in chronic myelogenous leukemia and relevance to treatment. *Leukemia*, 7: 1683–721.

Coulie, P. G., Lehmann, F., Lethe, B., Herman, J., Lurquin, C., Andrawiss, M. and Boon, T. (1995). A mutated intron sequence codes for an antigenic peptide recognized by cytolytic T lymphocytes on a human melanoma. *Proceedings of the National Academy of Sciences of the United States of America*, 92: 7976–80.

Denekamp, J. (1984). Vasculature as a target for tumor therapy. *Progress in Applied Microcirculation*, 4: 28–38.

Deweindt, C., Kerckaer, J-P., Tilly, H., Quief, S., Nguyen, V. C. and Basterd, C. (1993). Cloning of a breakpoint cluster region at band 3q27 involved in human non-Hodgkin's lymphoma. *Genes Chromosomes and Cancer*, 8: 149.

Dvir, A., Milner, Y., Chomsky, O. et al. (1991). The inhibition of EGF-dependent proliferation of keratinocytes by tyrphostin tyrosine kinase blockers. *Journal of Cell Biology*, 113: 857–65.

Evans, G., Harrington, E., Fanidi, A., Land, H., Amati, B. and Bennett, M. (1994). Integrated control of cell proliferation and cell death by the c-myc oncogene. *Philosophical Transactions of the Royal Society of London Biological Sciences*, 345: 269–75.

Feng, J., Funk, W. D., Wang, S-S., Weinrich, S. L., Avilion, A. A., Chiu, C-P., Adams, R. R., Chang, E., Allsopp, R. C., Yu, J., Le, S., West, M. D., Harley, C. B., Andrews, W. H., Greider, C. W. and Villeponteau, B. (1995). The RNA component of human telomerase. *Science*, 269: 1236–70.

Fishel, R. and Kolodner, R. D. (1995). Identification of mismatch repair genes and their role in the development of cancer. *Current Opinion in Genetics and Development*, 5: 382–95.

Folkman, J. (1995a). Angiogenesis in cancer, vascular, rheumatoid and other disease. *Nature Medicine*, 1: 27–31.

Folkman, J. (1995b). Angiogenesis inhibitors generated by tumors. *Molecular Medicine*, 1: 120–2.

Folkman, J. (1995c). The influence of angiogenesis research on management of patients with breast cancer. *European Journal of Cancer*, 31: 1101–4.

Fujiwara, T., Grimm, E. A., Mukhopadhyay, T. et al. (1994). Induction of chemosensitivity in human lung cancer cell in vivo by adenovirus-mediated transfer of wild type p53 gene. *Cancer Research*, **54**: 2287–91.

Gewirtz, A. M. (1993). Potential therapeutic applications of antisene oligodeoxynucleotides in the treatment of chronic myelogenous leukemia. *Leukemia and Lymphoma*, **11**: 131–7.

Gibbs, J. B. (1992). Pharmacological probes of Ras function. *Seminars in Cancer Biology*, **3**: 383–90.

Gibbs, J. B., Oliff, A. and Kohl, N. E. (1994). Farnesyltransferase inhibitors: ras research yields a potential cancer therapeutic. *Cell*, **77**: 175–8.

Golub, T. R., Barker, G. F., Luvett, M. and Gilliland, D. G. (1994). Fusion of PDGF receptor to a novel ets-like gene, tel, in chronic myelomonocytic leukemia with t(5;12) chromosomal translocation. *Cell*, **77**: 307–16.

Gutierrez, M. I., Bhatia, K. and Barriga, F. (1992). Molecular epidemiology of Burkitt's lymphoma from South America: differences in breakpoint location and Epstein–Barr virus association from tumors in other world regions. *Blood*, **79**: 3261–6.

Gutierrez, M. I., Judde, J-G., Magrath, I. T. and Bhatia, K. G. (1996). Switching viral latency to viral lysis: a novel therapeutic approach for Epstein Barr virus-associated neoplasia. *Cancer Research*, **56**: 969–72.

Hall, A. (1992). Signal transduction through small GTPases – a tale of two GAPS. *Cell*, **69**: 389–91.

Harris, C. C. (1992). Molecular basis of multistage carcinogenesis. In *Multistage Carcinogenesis*, ed. C. C. Harris, S. Hirohashi, N. Ito, H. C. Pitot, T. Sugimura, M. Terada and J. Yokota, pp. 3–19. CRC Press, Boca Raton, Florida; Tokyo, Japan Science Society Press.

Hartwell, L. H. and Kastan, M. B. (1994). Cell cycle control and cancer. *Science*, **266**: 1821–8.

Hawkins, M. J. (1995). Clinical trials of antiangiogenic agents. *Current Opinions in Oncology*, **7**: 90–3.

Hu, G., Liu, W., Hanania, E. G., Fu, S., Wang, T. and Deisseroth, A. B. (1995). Suppression of tumorigenesis by transcription units expressing the antisene E6 and E7 messenger RNA (mRNA) for the transforming proteins of the human papilloma virus and the sense mRNA for the retinoblastoma gene in cervical carcinoma cells. *Cancer Gene Therapy*, **2**: 19–32.

Huang, H. J., Yee, J. K., Shew, J. Y. et al. (1988). Suppression of the neoplastic phenotype by replacement of the RB gene in human cancer cells. *Science*, **242**: 1563–6.

Huber, B. E., Austin, E. A., Good, S. S. et al. (1993). In vivo antitumor activity of 5-fluorocytosine on human colorectal carcinoma cells genetically modified to express cytosine deaminase. *Cancer Research*, **53**: 4619–26.

Huber, H. E., Koblan, K. S. and Heimbrook, D. C. (1994). Protein–protein interactions as therapeutic targets for cancer. *Current Medicinal Chemistry*, **1**: 13–34.

Ingber, D., Fujita, T., Kishimoto, S., Sudo, K., Kanamaru, T., Bern, H. et al. (1990). Synthetic analogs of fumagillin that inhibit angiogenesis and suppress tumor growth. *Nature*, **348**: 555–7.

Judde, J-G., Spangler, G., Magrath, T. and Bhatia, K. (1996). Use of Epstein–Barr virus nuclear antigen-1 in targeted therapy of EBV associated neoplasia. *Cancer Research*, **56**: 969–72.

Kim, N. W., Piatyszek, M. A., Prowse, K. R., Harley, C. B., West, M. D., Ho, P. L. C., Coviello, G. M., Wright, W. E., Weinrich, S. L. and Shay, J. W. (1994). Specific association of human telomerase activity with immortal cells and cancer. *Science*, **266**: 2011–15.

Klein, E. and Klein, G. (1964). Antigenic properties of lymphomas induced by the Moloney agents. *Journal of the National Cancer Institute*, **32**: 547.

Klein, G. and Klein, E. (1985). Evolution of tumours and the impact of molecular oncology. *Nature*, **315**: 190–5.

Klinken, S. P., Alexander, W. S. and Adams, J. M. (1988). Hemopoietic lineage switch: v-raf oncogene converts Eμ-myc transgenic B cells into macrophages. *Cell*, **53**: 857–67.

Kuamble, T., Sohma, Y., Kayama, T., Yoshimoto, T. and Yamamoto, T. (1992). Amplification of PDGFR, a gene lacking an exon coding for a portion of the extracellular region in a primary brain tumor of glial origin. *Oncogene*, **7**: 627–33.

Liebermann, D. A. and Hoffman, B. (1994). Differentiation primary response genes and proto-oncogenes as positive and negative regulators of terminal hematopoietic cell differentiation. *Stem Cells*, **12**: 352–69.

Luders, G., Kohnlein, W., Sorg, C. and Bruggen, J. (1985). Selective toxicity of neocarzinostatin–monoclonal antibody conjugates to the antigen-bearing human melanoma cell line in vitro. *Cancer Immunology and Immunotherapy*, **20**: 85–90.

Magrath, T. (1990). The pathogenesis of Burkitt's lymphoma. *Advances in Cancer Research*, **55**: 133–270.

Marasca, R., Longo, G., Luppi, M., Barozzi, P. and Torelli, G. (1994). Double p53 point mutation in extramedullary blast crisis of chronic myelogenous leukemia. *Leukemia and Lymphoma*, **16**: 171–5.

Martiny-Baron, G. and Marme, D. (1995). VEGF-mediated tumour angiogenesis: a new target for cancer therapy. *Current Opinion in Biotechnology*, **6**: 675–80.

McManaway, M. E., Neckers, L. M., Loke, S. L. et al. (1990). Tumor-specific inhibition of lymphoma growth by an antisene oligodeoxynucleotide. *Lancet*, **335**: 808–11.

Morris, S. W., Kirsten, M. N., Valentine, M. B., Dittmer, K. G., Shapiro, D. N., Slatman, D. L. and Look, A. T. (1994). Fusion of a kinase gene, ALK, to a nucleolar protein gene, NPM, in non-Hodgkin's lymphoma. *Science*, **263**: 1281–4.

Murakami, Y., Mizuno, S., Hori, M. et al. (1988). Reversal of transformed phenotypes by herbimycin A in sarc oncogene expressed in rat fibroblasts. *Cancer Research*, **48**: 1587–90.

Nowell, P. C. (1976). The clonal evolution of tumor cell populations. *Science*, **194**: 23–8.

Okuda, T., van Deursen, J. V., Hiebert, S. W. et al. (1996). AML-1, the target of multiple chromosomal translocations in human leukemia, is essential for normal fetal liver hematopoiesis. *Cell*, **84**: 321–30.

Old, L. J. (1981). Cancer immunology: the search for specificity – G. H. A. Clowes Memorial lecture. *Cancer Research*, **41**: 361–75.

O'Neil, K. T. and Hoess, R. H. (1995). Phage display: protein engineering by directed evolution. *Current Opinion in Structural Biology*, **5**: 443–9.

Perrouault, L., Asseline, U., Rivalle, C. et al. (1990). Sequence specific artificial photoinduced endonucleases based on triple helix-forming oligonucleotides. *Nature*, **344**: 358–60.

Rabbits, T. H. (1991). Translocations, master genes and differences between the origins of acute and chronic leukemias. *Cell*, **67**: 641–4.

Radman, M., Matic, I., Halliday, J. A. and Taddei, F. (1995). Editing DNA replication and recombination by mismatch repair: from bacterial genetics to mechanisms of predisposition to cancer in humans. *Philosophical Transactions of the Royal Society of London Biological Sciences*, **347**: 97–103.

Rak, J. W., St Croix, B. D. and Kerbel, R. S. (1995). Consequences of angiogenesis for tumor progression, metastasis and cancer therapy. *Anticancer Drugs*, **6**: 3–18.

Rovira, A., Urbano-Ispizua, A., Cervantes, F., Rozman, M., Vives-Corrons, J. L., Montserrat, E. and Rozman, C. (1995). P53 tumor suppressor gene in chronic myelogenous leukemia: a sequential study. *Annals of Hematology*, **70**: 129–33.

Santoso, J. T., Tang, D. C., Lane, S. B., Hung, J., Reed, D. J., Muller, C. Y., Carbone, D. P., Lucci, J. A., Miller, D. S. and Mathis, J. M. (1995). Adenovirus-based p53 gene therapy in ovarian cancer. *Gynecological Oncology*, **59**: 171–8.

Satoh, T. and Kaziro, Y. (1992). Ras in signal transduction. *Cancer Biology*, **3**: 169–77.

Schumacher, T. N., Mayr, L. M., Minor, D. L., Milhollen, M. A., Burgess, M. W. and Kim, P. S. (1996). Identification of D-peptide ligands through mirror-image phase display. *Science*, **271**: 1854–7.

Skorski, T., Skorska, M. N., Barletta, C. et al. (1993). Highly efficient elimination of philadelphia leukemic cells by exposure to bcr/abl antisene oligodeoxynucleotides combined with mafosfamide. *Journal of Clinical Investigation*, **92**: 194–202.

Smetsers, T. F., Skorski, T., Van de Locht, L. T. et al. (1994). Antisense BCR-ARL oligonucleotides induce apoptosis in the philadelphia chromosome-positive cell line 13V173. *Leukemia*, **8**: 129–40.

Stein, C. A. (1992). Anti-sense oligodeoxynucleotides – promises and pitfalls. *Leukemia*, **6**: 967–74.

Stein, C. A. and Cohen, J. S. (1988). Oligodeoxynucleotides as inhibitors of gene expression: a review. *Cancer Research*, **48**: 2659–68.

Suter, L., Bruggen, J., Brocker, E. B. and Sorg, C. (1985). A tumor-associated antigen expressed in melanoma cells with lower malignant potential. *International Journal of Cancer*, **35**: 787–91.

Szczylik, C. T., Skorski, N. C., Nicolaides, I. et al. (1991). Selective inhibition of leukemia cell proliferation by BCR-ABL antisense oligodeoxynucleotides. *Science*, **253**: 562–5.

Teicher, B. A. (1995). Angiogenesis and cancer metastases: therapeutic approaches. *Critical Reviews in Oncology and Hematology*, **20**: 9–39.

Van Pel, A., De Plaen, E., Lurquin, C., Van den Eynde, B., Lethe, B., Hainaut, P., Lemoine, C. and Boon, T. (1988). Identification of genes encoding T cell defined tumor-antigens. *Princess Takamatsu Symposium*, **19**: 255–63.

Vogelstein, B. and Kinzler, K. W. (1993). The multistep nature of cancer. *Trends in Genetics*, **9**: 138–41.

Wang, C. and Huang, L. (1987). Ph-sensitive immunoliposomes mediate target-cell-specific delivery and controlled expression of a foreign gene in mouse. *Proceedings of the National Academy of Sciences of the United States of America*, **84**: 7851–5.

Yang, J. H., Cedergren, R. and Nada-Ginard, B. (1994). Catalytic activity of an RNA domain derived from the U6-U4 RNA complex. *Science*, **263**: 77–81.

Yates, J., Warren, N., Reisman, D. and Sugden, B. (1984). A cis-acting element from the Epstein–Barr viral genome that permits stable replication of recombinant plasmids in latently infected cells. *Proceedings of the National Academy of Sciences of the United States of America*, **83**: 3806–10.

Ye, B. H., Lista, F., LoCoco, F., Knowles, D. M., Offit, K., Chaganti, R. S. K. and Dalla-Favera, R. (1993). Alterations of a zn-finger encoding gene BCL-6 in diffuse large cell lymphoma. *Science*, **262**: 747.

Yuan, C. J., Jakes, S. and Elliot, S. (1990). A rationale for the design of an inhibitor of tyrosyl kinase. *Journal of Biological Chemotherapy*, **265**: 2255.

3

Vectors for cancer gene therapy

PREM SETH

In recent years there has been a dramatic increase in developing gene therapy approaches for the treatment of cancer. In principle, gene therapy involves the transfer of foreign genetic material into a patient in an effort to treat a particular disease (Mulligan, 1993). The two events which have permitted the formulation of the concept of cancer gene therapy are the new understanding of the molecular mechanisms underlying oncogenesis and the development of the DNA-delivery vehicles, or vectors. It was initially thought that successful gene therapy would require that pre-existing defects be corrected in every cancer cell. However, in recent years it has become clear that a high level of transient gene expression in even a limited number of the target cells could also be potentially beneficial. Many approaches to cancer gene therapy have been proposed, and many viral and nonviral vectors have been utilized. The purpose of this chapter is to describe the biology, construction and unique characteristics of some of the commonly used vectors, and some of the pre-clinical studies that have been performed with them. The problems associated with these vectors, and future considerations pertaining to vector development for the gene therapy of cancer are also discussed. The clinical protocols utilizing these vectors are discussed in various chapters throughout the book.

The use of recombinant vectors for cancer gene therapy

Our understanding that cancer is a multistage process that involves not only the molecular alterations in the malignant cells themselves, such as loss of tumor suppressor genes, but also additional immunological defects leading to the inability of the immune system to destroy the cancer cells, has contributed a great deal to devising the various approaches to cancer gene therapy. Before attempting to initiate a cancer gene therapy program, one needs to determine which gene therapy approach is best suited for the disease in question. Some of the approaches that have been explored to date are described below.

1. Vectors expressing genes whose protein product would kill and/or cause the growth-arrest of the tumor cells. Examples of such genes are toxin genes (*Pseudomonas* exotoxin), tumor suppressors (p53), and cyclin kinase inhibitors (p21/WAF1, p27/Kip1). Such vectors can be directly injected into the tumor masses, targeted to tumor cells or can be used ex vivo for killing tumor cells, for example for bone marrow purging before autologous bone marrow transplantation. The efficacies of many of these gene therapy agents will, however, be dependent upon the fraction of tumor cells transduced.

2. Vectors expressing suicide genes whose protein product will kill the cells when simultaneously exposed to small molecular weight drugs (the enzyme/prodrug approach). An example is the use of vector-containing bacterial cytosine deaminase in combination with the systemic delivery of 5-fluorocytosine (5-FC) which is converted by cytosine deaminase to 5-fluorouracil (5-FU), a cytotoxic drug. Another example is the use of herpes simplex virus thymidine kinase (HSV TK) in combination with gancyclovir, which produces phosphorylated gancyclovir as the toxic species. This approach of cell killing is further mediated by the 'bystander effects' of the toxic product whereby adjacent cells are killed by the activated drug. These vectors can be injected directly into the tumor mass, used ex vivo to kill tumor cells, or, theoretically, delivered systemically and targeted to tumor cells.

3. Vectors expressing genes that will inactivate the dominant oncogenes, for example vectors expressing antisense or ribozymes directed against the *ras* (or other) oncogene. This approach can be also targeted against the tumors in vivo or for killing cells ex vivo.

4. Vectors expressing genes that enhance or induce an antitumor immune response. This can be accomplished by using cell-based cancer vaccines, in which case the individual can be vaccinated with autologous tumor cells expressing vector-mediated cytokines – interleukin-2 (IL-2), IL-4, IL-12, tumor necrosis factor (TNF), interferon-γ, granulocyte macrophage colony stimulating factor (GM-CSF); genes that have immunostimulatory activity – allogenic major histocompatability complex antigens, adhesion molecules; or T-cell costimulatory molecules such as B7.1 and B7.2. Vectors expressing cytokines and immunomodulators can also be directly injected into the tumor but are likely to be most useful when injected at a distant site, giving the maximal probability of exciting an immune response.

5. Vector-mediated gene transfer to T lymphocytes or dendritic cells that will enhance their antitumor effector activity. For example, tumor-infiltrating lymphocytes can be transduced with vectors expressing genes encoding cytokines, such as TNF-α, to induce antitumor activity. Similarly, vectors can be used to express variable regions of tumor-specific monoclonal antibodies to recognize and kill the tumor cells.

6. Vectors whose protein products are capable of inhibiting tumor angiogenesis, e.g. by downregulating vascular endothelial growth factor expression. This can be conducted by injecting the vectors directly into the tumor or targeting to vascular endothelial cells lining the blood vessels of the tumor.

7. Vector-mediated gene transfer of drug-resistant genes that can be transduced into hematopoietic stem cells to increase their resistance to cytotoxic drugs. The most widely studied gene for this purpose is the multidrug-resistant-1 gene (*MDR-1*). Bone marrow cells expressing MDR should be more resistant to conventional chemotherapy and hence allow patients to receive higher doses of chemotheraupitic agents. Success with this approach will be dependent upon the expansion of MDR-transduced cells when exposed to drugs to which *MDR-1* expression induces resistance as well as sensitivity of the tumor cells to the same drugs.

Choice of vectors

There are essentially two major classes of vectors: viral based and nonviral based. Because viruses have evolved a natural mechanism to deliver their genomes into cells, they are excellent vectors to deliver foreign DNA, if inserted properly into the virion particles. Nonviral vectors can also enhance delivery of the nucleic acids to the cells, usually by binding to the cell membrane or a specific receptor. Before a particular vector is selected, it is important to understand what is expected from the vector. Some of the important considerations for selecting particular vectors are described in Table 3.1.

Viral vectors

Much of the work on gene therapy has been conducted using retroviruses, adenoviruses and adeno-associated viruses. However, in recent years, several other viral vectors, including some chimeric vectors, have been described and will be discussed here. While the choice of vector will depend upon the

44 *Prem Seth*

Table 3.1. *Important considerations for selecting the vector*

- What are the target cells? These could be tumor cells or host cells such as T cells or bone marrow cells. One needs to know the precise developmental nature of the target cells, i.e., whether these cells are of epithelial origin, hematopoietic stem cells, neuronal cells, skin cells etc.
- Are the target cells undergoing active mitotic division or are they quiescent? It might be beneficial to alter the mitotic state of the cells before/during gene transfer.
- How many cells target cells need to be targeted for successful gene therapy? In some instances, targeting a few cells might be enough, whereas in other instances, transfer to a larger population (even 100%) may be essential.
- How will the vector be delivered? Vectors can be administered systemically, injected into the tumor or at sites distant from the tumor or can be applied ex vivo.
- Is short-term expression of the heterologous protein enough, or is long-term production of the protein essential for an efficacious result?
- Are there pre-existing antibodies to the vector of choice that could influence the outcome of gene therapy?
- What factors might interfere or produce harmful effects during the treatment? One needs to be particularly aware of the situations in which nonreplicating vectors can be easily converted into replicating forms that could potentially have serious harmful effects.

experimental or clinical setting, it is conceivable that several vectors would represent reasonable choice. In such a circumstance, other general considerations listed in Table 3.2 will play a role in the selection of the optimal vector.

Retroviral vectors

Molecular biology of retroviruses

In many of the initial studies of viral-mediated gene transfer, retroviruses have been used as vectors. The main reason for this is that upon entry of the retroviruses into the cells, the genomic proviral sequences of retroviruses can integrate into the host genome such that stable transfection is achieved (i.e., the vector is not readily lost from the cell). One of the most widely studied vectors is the Moloney murine leukemia virus (MoMuLV) (Cone and Mulligan, 1992). This retrovirus is composed of a double-stranded RNA genome consisting of 5' long terminal repeats (LTR), which include sequences responsible for virus integration and regulation of the transcription of viral genes. Adjacent to the 5' LTR is region (–P) where the tRNA primer binds and reverse transcription is initiated. Next to this are splice donor and encapsidation sequences, *gag, pol* and *env* genes that encode for the viral structural proteins: ribonucleoprotein core (*gag*); protease, reverse transcriptase/RNaseH, and

Table 3.2. *Desirable features of recombinant viral vectors*

- Should be relatively easy to generate and grow to high titers in the laboratory.
- Should be free of any contamination of wild-type vector that might produce harmful effects. The potential severity of this problem may vary for the different vectors.
- The packaging capacity of the vector should be large enough to accommodate commonly used cDNAs. Sometimes it is desirable to have more than one transgene expression in the same vector, or to use large genomic sequences.
- Administration of the vector into the desired site should be feasible and the vector should be able to target the tissue of interest. Although most large vectors are designed to be administered locally, there should be potential to deliver them systemically.
- Vector-mediated gene expression should be at a high enough level for the desirable length of time. This is particularly relevant for those vectors that mediate short-term gene expression.
- Should be able to modify vector tropism and tissue specificity if needed.
- Viral-mediated expression of the genes should be possible in dividing and nondividing cells.
- Vector should have minimum undesirable immune responses.
- Administration of the vector should not produce any serious harmful effects.
- Repeat administration of the vector (if needed) should be possible.
- In the event of any harmful effects, should be possible to stop the vector treatment immediately and the subsequent expression of the foreign gene.
- Since gene therapy to only somatic cells is currently being considered, the vector should not reach the gonadal tissues, and if it does, should not be able to integrate into reproductive cells.

integrase enzymes (*pol*); and the envelope glycoproteins (*env*). Between the terminus of the *env* gene and the 3' LTR is a purine-rich region that serves as a site for the initiation of plus strand cDNA synthesis (+P) during reverse transcription. The 3' LTR includes all of the information present in the 5'-LTR, and also provides polyadenylation signals (Coffin, 1996).

Life cycle of retroviruses

Retroviral entry into cells is initiated by the binding of the *env*-encoded glycoprotein to its cellular receptor. The host range of the virion infection is dependent upon the type of glycoprotein encoded by the *env* gene. Four different proteins determine whether the retrovirus is ecotropic, amphotropic, xenotropic or polytropic (Battini, Heard and Danos, 1992). The cellular receptors for retroviruses have been reported to be either cationic amino acid transporters or a phosphate carrier (Wang et al., 1991; Kavanaugh et al., 1994). After binding to its receptor, the virus envelope fuses with the plasma membrane. Alternatively, virus may enter the endosome and fuse with the endosome membrane. This results in the release of the virion content into the cytosol. After the virus is uncoated, one of the RNA strands is transcribed by the reverse transcriptase, resulting in the formation of DNA–RNA hybrids. An RNase activity associated with the reverse transcriptase is responsible for the digestion of the RNA strand, and the DNA strand is then replicated by the retroviral DNA polymerase. The resulting double-stranded DNA is finally incorporated into random sites in the host genome by the retroviral integrase enzyme (Coffin, 1996).

Generation of recombinant retroviruses

To generate recombinant retroviral vectors, the genes *gag*, *pol* and *env*, which are required for viral replication, are replaced by the cDNA of choice (up to 8 kb) in a vector that also contains the packaging signals. Cell lines that constitutively express the *gag*, *pol* and *env* genes of MoMuLV are generated in parallel. By expressing viral proteins, these cell lines provide the necessary helper function for the propagation of retrovirus vector particles that lack the genes needed for viral replication (Danos and Mulligan, 1988; Markowitz, Goff and Bank, 1988). The vector containing the foreign cDNA is then transfected into the helper cell line, resulting in the production of recombinant replication-incompetent retroviral particles (Figure 3.1). If a selectable marker such as *neo*^{R} is also introduced in the vector, the individual clones of the producer cell lines can be grown in the presence of neomycin, and used directly for gene-transfer experiments. Alternatively, one can use the supernatants from the producer cell lines, which contain the recombinant retroviral particles. Viral particles produced from such cells cannot reproduce in the normal host, but can carry the foreign gene into the host cell.

Features of recombinant retroviral vectors, and recent improvements in vector development

Since retroviruses are capable of integrating into the host genome, they are excellent vectors when the long-term expression of the foreign gene is needed. One of the concerns in using recombinant retroviruses for gene therapy, however, has been the risk of accidentally producing wild-type retrovirus that could lead to virus replication and, potentially, public safety concern (Donahue et al., 1992). Despite this theoretical risk, clinical use of retroviral vectors so far has been found to be safe with the current generation of packaging cell lines.

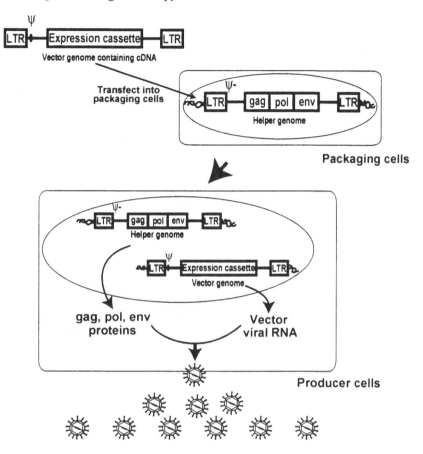

Recombinant Retroviral Particles

Fig. 3.1. *Construction of recombinant retroviruses.* The gag, pol and env sequences of MoMuLV encoding for structural and catalytic proteins are replaced by the cDNA of interest. However, the packaging signal is retained in this recombinant viral genome. The plasmid DNA is transfected into a packaging cell line stably expressing gag, pol and env proteins (helper genome devoid of Ψ (packaging signal). These cells can package the viral RNA transcripts because they contain the Ψ signal. Producer cells producing recombinant retroviral particles or cell supernatants containing the retroviral particles can be used as a source of recombinant retroviruses.

Another potential problem associated with retroviruses results from their random integration into the host chromosome. This could result in deleterious effects such as the activation of certain proto-oncogenes (by a mechanism known as insertional mutagenesis, in which viral LTR activates certain adjacent genes), or suppression of other tumor suppressor genes (e.g., by disruption of the gene or its regulatory elements). Moreover, the expression of the foreign gene can be affected by the insertion site of the provirus in the host chromosomes as well as by interference between viral and host promoters; and hence the expression of the transgene in individual cells can be variable.

Retroviruses have, until recently, been produced in relatively low titers (10^6–10^7 particles/ml) of the virus, a problem which can be compounded by the low concentration of recombinants in the viral supernatants produced. However, modified retroviral vectors have been designed, based on the observation that the viral sequences necessary for efficient packaging of the retroviral RNA extends into the *gag* gene. These retroviral vectors have much better packaging efficiency (Bender et al., 1987). Another way to increase the production of retroviral proteins, and hence to increase the titer, is by using packaging plasmids containing the sequences that lead to amplification of the plasmids in packaging cell lines (Takahara, Hamada and Housman, 1992). Another way to increase the copy number of the proviral particles is by coculturing producer cells that release viral particles with different tropisms, commonly referred to as the 'ping pong' method (Lynch and Miller, 1991: Hoatlin et al., 1995; Miller and Chen, 1996). In addition, other helper-free systems that yield high titers of retroviruses have also been described recently (Naviaux et al., 1996), and progress has been made in the optimization of growth medium conditions.

Whatever the viral titer, a potential barrier to effective cell transduction by MoMuLV is the requirement of cell division for provirus integration (Miller, Adam and Miller, 1990). This problem can be overcome in some circumstances by using lenti viruses (described below) that are capable of integrating into nondividing cells. A similar limitation in the use of retroviral-mediated gene therapy is the limited host range of these viruses. This difficulty has been largely surmounted by the use of 'pseudotype' retroviral vectors grown in packaging cell lines that express the envelope proteins of the viruses with a different or broader range (Yee et al., 1994). For example, the env protein of MoMuLV has been replaced by the G protein of vesicular stomatitis virus (VSV). VSV G protein has a much broader host specificity because it can enter the cells via receptors such as phosphatidyl serine (Ory, Neugeboren and Mulligan, 1996). Of course, for gene therapy, a rather narrow host range (ideally, confined to tumor cells) is preferable. Since retroviruses do not target specific cell types, attempts have been made to modify their tissue tropism via genetically modifying the viral envelope to include specific ligand-binding moieties or by linking the envelope with single-chain antibodies that bind to specific cellular membrane proteins (Gunzburg and Salmons, 1996; Somia, Zoppe and Verma, 1995; Cosset and Russell, 1996). Recombinant retroviruses have also been constructed ultizing cell-specific promoters such as carcino-embryonic antigen (CEA) and tyrosinase promoters (Vile et al., 1994, 1995, 1996; Richards, Austin and Huber, 1995).

Finally, the use of retroviruses in-vivo is limited by inactivation by serum complements. Interestingly, however, retroviruses produced by the packaging cells of human origin are much more resistant to inactivation by complement (Pensiero et al., 1996).

Preclinical studies using recombinant retroviruses

Since retroviruses can infect epithelial as well as hematopoietic cells, they have been extensively used as gene vectors. For gene-therapy purposes investigators have used either the producer (packaging) cell lines themselves or purified retroviral vectors capable of expressing recombinant retroviruses. Retroviral vectors expressing the tumor suppressor gene *p53* and *K-ras* antisense have been shown to induce cytotoxicity to tumor cells (Zhang et al. 1993; Cai et al., 1993). Retroviral vectors expressing suicide genes *HSV TK*, and *E. coli* cytosine deaminase have been constructed. These vectors are capable of converting the prodrugs gancyclovir and 5-FC into the cytotoxic compounds gancyclovir phosphate and 5-FU to kill cancer cells (Ram et al., 1994b; Trinh et al., 1995). In these experiments, in-vitro toxicity to various cancer cells as well as in-vivo efficacy in inhibiting tumor growth in murine models have been demonstrated. Retroviruses have also been used to express cytokines such as IL-2, GM-CSF and immunomodulator B7.1 in tumor cells. Similarly, IL-2, TNF-α, and tumor-associated antigens have been transferred, using retroviral vectors, to T cells for immunotherapy purposes (Dranoff et al., 1993; Hwu et al., 1993; Sanda et al., 1994; Ram et al., 1994a; Mule et al., 1996; Simons et al., 1997). Retroviruses have been used for gene-marking clinical trials. For example, the *neo*[R] gene has been used to mark bone marrow cells and T cells (Dilloo et al., 1996; Bunnell et al., 1997) in order to follow the fate of the marked cells after infusion of the transduced cells into the animals or patients. Finally, retroviruses containing multidrug resistant genes have been used to transduce murine bone marrow cells. Upon subsequent transfer of these transduced cells to the animals, much higher doses of chemotherapeutic drugs could be tolerated, thus establishing the validity of the concept that chemoresistance of myelopoietic cells can be induced into cells, which then preferentially survive the administration of chemotherapeutic drugs (Licht et al., 1995).

Based on these preclinical experiments, it can be concluded that retroviral vectors are, at the very least, useful tools for establishing the principles of

cancer gene therapy. Currently, many recombinant retroviral vectors are being
used for Phase I clinical trials.

Adenoviral vectors

Molecular biology of adenoviruses

Adenoviruses are DNA-containing, nonenveloped viruses. About 47 human
serotypes have been isolated, which are classified into six subgroups (groups
A to F). Adenoviruses generally infect the differentiated cells of ocular tissue,
the upper and lower respiratory tracts and the gastrointestinal tract. The two
adenoviruses most commonly used for constructing recombinant vectors are
Ad2 and Ad5, both of which belong to group C. These virions are icosahedral
in shape, about 70–100 nm diameter, and consist of proteins and DNA. There
is a capsid composed of seven known structural proteins and a core that has
four proteins bound to the viral DNA (Shenk, 1996). The adenovirus genome
consists of a single piece of linear double-stranded DNA, approximately 36 kb
long and flanked by two short, inverted terminal repeats. The genome is
composed of various transcriptional regions that include an early region (E1
through E4), two delayed early units (IX and 1Va2), a late region (L1 through
L5), and VA regions. The E1 region encodes two proteins, E1a and E1b,
which have many functions including the regulation of other viral transcriptional units, and inducing the host cells to enter S phase. E2 encodes three
proteins, including a DNA-binding protein, DNA polymerase, and the terminal
binding proteins responsible for adenoviral DNA replication. Proteins encoded
by the E3 region are involved in mechanisms used by the virus to evade the
immune system. E4 region proteins are involved in viral transcription, DNA
replication, mRNA transport, and in turning off host protein synthesis. After
the onset of the viral replication, the major late promoter located at 16 map
units drives much of the subsequent viral transcription. Late viral proteins
derived from region L1–L5 encode structural proteins, including capsid proteins hexon, penton base and penton fiber. These capsid proteins facilitate
the entry of adenoviruses into the cells (Shenk, 1996).

Life cycle of adenoviruses

Adenoviruses enter cells by receptor-mediated endocytosis (Seth et al., 1986).
The virus binds to the cell receptor through its fiber protein. Molecular cloning
of the adenovirus receptors has suggested that they are members of a family
of receptors used by Coxsackie B viruses (Bergelson et al., 1997). Besides the

adenovirus primary receptors, integrin proteins may function as the secondary receptors for adenovirus. After binding to its receptor, adenovirus–receptor complexes appear in clathrin-coated pits which internalize as endocytic vesicles called endosomes. Adenovirus can enter the cytoplasm by rupturing the membrane of the endosome. Rupture appears to be a consequence of the low pH of the endosome, which induces a conformational change in the viral penton base such that virus can bind to the inner membrane of the endosome (Seth, 1994a). It has been proposed that this causes the activation of a membrane-bound ATPase, which results in the build-up of osmotic pressure inside the endosome, with resultant rupture at the point of contact (Figure 3.2). Adenoviruses then traverse towards the nucleus and, by an unknown mechanism, release their genome into the nucleus. Immediately after entry into the nucleus, viral early genes (*E1*, *E2*, *E4*) are transcribed, and the protein products help in adenoviral DNA replication, and late transcription. For adenovirus replication to proceed, adenovirus proteins (E1a, E1b-55 kDa proteins) induce cells into S-phase, and E1b-19 kDa protein prevents the host cells undergoing apoptosis. Once viral DNA replication is under way, host protein mRNA transport and protein sythesis are shut off by the early gene proteins E1B-55 kDa protein, E4orf6, VA RNA and tripartite leader. Once the late genes that encode for viral structural proteins (hexon, penton base, fiber) are expressed, assembly of the virus takes place in the nucleus, and within 24 hours of viral entry into the cells, new virion particles can be detected. Several thousand viral particles can be produced per cell. Eventually, cells die of necrosis, and the virion particles are released from the cell (Shenk, 1996).

Generation of the recombinant adenoviruses

Recombinant adenoviruses can be readily generated by replacing E1 and E3 sequences in adenovirus DNA by the foreign cDNA. Because E1 sequences are required for viral replication, replacing them with heterologous DNA sequences generates recombinant adenoviruses that are replication defective. To generate recombinant adenoviruses, a cDNA of choice coupled to an appropriate promoter is cloned into a shuttle vector that provides the left adenovirus inverted terminal repeat (ITR), origin of replication, E1a enhancer, encapsidation signals and adenovirus homologous recombination sequences downstream of the E1 region. Adenovirus genome can be obtained either from restriction-enzyme-digested adenovirus genome, e.g., using a Cla1 site located near the left end of the adenovirus genome dl327 (Stratford-Perricaudet et al., 1992). Alternatively, plasmid DNA containing the various versions of the adenovirus genome vectors (e.g., pJM17, pBHG10) can be

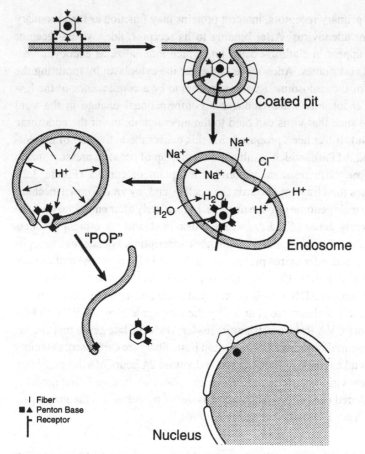

Fig. 3.2. *Model of adenovirus entry and vesicle disruption.* Adenovirus binds to a cell surface receptor and moves into a coated pit. Soon thereafter, it appears in endosome. Low pH of the endosome causes the penton base protein to undergo a conformational change (from ▲ to ■), as a result of which penton base acquires amphiphilic characteristics that enable it to interact with the membrane of the endosome. Endosome, which is distended as a result of osmotic pressure, ruptures at the point where adenovirus penetrates the membrane.

used (Bett et al., 1994). The large genomic adenoviral DNA and the shuttle vector are then cotransfected into a packaging cell line 293, which is an adenovirus transformed cell line which provides the E1 proteins in *trans*. Homologous recombination results in the generation of a recombinant adenovirus devoid of E1 sequences (Figure 3.3). Viral individual plaques are then picked, screened for the absense of E1 and the presence of the transgene, and then grown in 293 cells. Using these methods, recombinant adenoviral vectors containing foreign genome of up to 7.5 kb can be generated. While E1-deleted

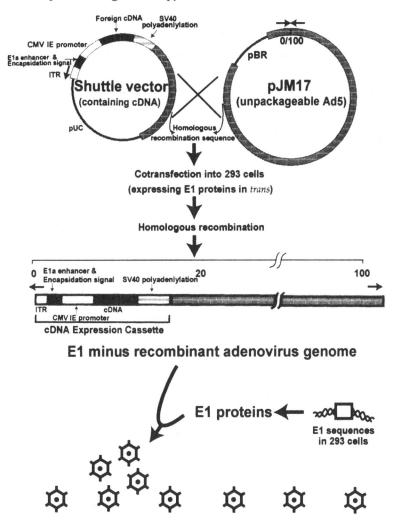

E1 minus recombinant adenovirus genome

Recombinant Adenoviral Particles

Fig. 3.3. *Construction of recombinant adenoviral vectors.* cDNA of interest is cloned into a shuttle vector that provides cDNA expression cassette (adenovirus ITR, E1 enhancer, adenovirus encapsidation signal, CMV promoter, and SV40 – a polyadenylation signal). Homologous recombination sequences are also cloned in this vector. Adenovirus genome (e.g., pJM17 shown in the figure) and the shuttle vector containing the cDNA are cotransfected in 293 cells. Intracellular homologous recombination between the two DNAs results in an E1⁻ recombinant genome; the numbers 0, 20, 100 represent the approximate map units. This recombinant genome is replication defective. However, in the presence of E1 proteins (provided in *trans* by 293 cells), the recombinant genome will replicate and form adenoviral particles.

first-generation adenoviral vectors are replication deficient, low-level viral protein expression has been detected in cells infected with these vectors. In an effort to minimize expression of viral proteins, recombinant adenoviral vectors containing either a ts mutant of E2a (Engelhardt, Litzky and Wilson, 1994) or deleted E4 sequences have been constructed (Armentano et al., 1995). Recombinant adenoviruses in which all viral genes have been deleted, such that they contain only viral ITR and contiguous packaging sequences, have also been constructed. The construction of these viral vectors requires the helper adenovirus from which E1 has been deleted. Alternatively, Cre-loxP recombination methods to generate recombinant adenoviruses have been employed. These cloning methods have permitted up to 35 kb of the foreign DNA to be cloned into adenoviruses (Parks et al., 1996; Fisher et al., 1996a; Hardy et al., 1997). Recombinant adenoviruses can be easily purified in a $CsCl_2$ gradient and stored, frozen, for an indefinite period of time.

Features of recombinant adenoviral vectors, and recent improvements in vector development

One of the reasons adenoviruses have become very popular vectors is the ease with which recombinant viruses can be generated and grown to very high titers (up to 10^{12} plaque-forming units (PFU)/ml in the laboratory). Adenoviruses have other characteristics that make them useful as vectors, including the very efficient receptor-mediated endocytosis and high level of gene transfer in cancer cells. This means that adenoviruses are suitable vectors in situations that require high-level gene expression for the short term. Because of their fairly large packaging capacity (up to 35 kb), adenoviruses can also be used to transfer larger genes than is possible with retroviruses. Another advantage of adenoviruses is that they can infect a variety of cell types and produce the heterologous protein of interest in dividing as well as nondividing cells. The use of adenoviruses as vectors is limited by the fact that they do not integrate into the host chromosomes or grow as episomal vectors, and they are degraded by the host. This results in a short-term expression of the transduced gene.

It has been suggested that immunological responses to adenoviruses may reduce the duration of expression of therapeutic gene (transgene). Both humoral immunity and cell-mediated immunity have been implicated in these immunological reactions (Dai et al., 1995). Although short-term gene expression by adenoviruses might still be sufficient for cancer gene therapy, there have been many attempts to reduce the immunogenicity of adenoviruses, thus permitting longer-term expression. Adenoviral vectors derived from E2a mutants and E4 deletion have been shown to be much less immunogenic, and to express transgene for a longer duration than those containing normal E2a and E4 sequences (Engelhardt, Litzky and Wilson, 1994; Armentano et al., 1995). The adenoviral vectors constructed by using minimum adenovirus sequences that lack immunological viral proteins are also expected to induce weaker immunological responses. Immunological rejection can be somewhat diminished by a quite different approach – use of cytokines such as IL-12 to inhibit the T-helper cells required for initiation of antiviral antibody production (Yang et al., 1996), or of cyclosporin to temporarily suppress the immune response (Kass-Eisler et al., 1996). Some investigators have utilized different adenoviral serotypes for serial administration of adenoviral vectors in an attempt to circumvent this problem (Kass-Eisler et al., 1996).

As with retroviruses, the possibility that replication-competent adenoviruses may be generated in patients must be considered. This could happen either spontaneously, during their propagation in a packaging cell line, or in the event that cells express transactivating factors such as IL-6 capable of substituting E1 functions (Higginbotham et al., unpublished; Deryckere and Burgert, 1996). Adenoviral vectors with longer deletions have been made in an attempt to lessen the risk.

Adenoviruses, like other viral vectors, lack cell and tissue specificity. Attempts have been made to target adenoviruses to specific cell types by coupling ligands or antibodies to the adenovirus capsid proteins. These modifications can be made to the viral coat proteins with or without modifying the fiber protein (Krasnykh et al., 1996). Alternatively, some investigators rendered transgene expression specific by using tissue-specific promoters such as CEA for the treatment of pancreatic and colonic cancers, mucin (MUC)-1 promoters for breast cancer cells, alpha-fetoprotein promoters for hepatocellular carcinoma, and tyrosinase promoter for melanoma, just to mention a few (Guo et al., 1996; Lan et al., 1996; Tanaka et al., 1996; Griscelli et al., 1997). Attempts have also been made to use inducible promoters such as the metallothionein promoter (Yajima et al., 1996).

Preclinical evaluation of recombinant adenoviral vectors

Numerous preclinical studies in which adenoviral vectors have been used are described in the literature. Adenoviruses expressing tumor suppressor genes such as *p53* have been shown to induce apoptosis in the cancer cells in vitro and in vivo (Katayose et al., 1995a; Nguyen et al., 1996; Spitz et al., 1996). Interestingly, cancers which are resistant to chemotherapeutic drugs are particularly sensitive to killing by a recombinant adenoviral vector expressing *p53* (Seth et al., 1997). Adenoviruses expressing inhibitors of cell cycle progression (p21/WAF1, p27/Kip1, p16/INK44A) have been shown to induce cell cycle arrest in vitro and in-vivo effects of inhibiting tumor growth in murine models (Katayose et al., 1995b; Craig et al., 1997). Adenoviruses expressing antisense and ribozymes to various cellular targets, including mutated *ras*, have been shown to have therapeutic effects on tumor growth in vivo (Kijima et al., 1995; Feng et al., 1995; Zhang, 1996). Adenoviral vectors expressing suicide genes such as *E. coli* cytosine deaminase, and HSV TK, when simultaneously treated with prodrugs 5-FC and gancyclovir respectively, have been shown to be effective in vitro, as well as inhibiting tumor growth in animal models (Elshami et al., 1996; Dong et al., 1996; Li et al., 1997).

Another area of active research, as with retroviral vectors, is to use recombinant adenoviruses to activate potentially tumor-directed immunological pathways. Adenoviruses expressing IL-2, IL-4, GM-CSF, B7.1, TNF-α, interferon-γ, and IL-12 have been successfully used to cause the expression of proteins in cells in vitro. Administration of these recombinant adenoviral vectors in vivo has been shown to result in the inhibition of tumor growth and/or vaccine effect (inhibition of tumor growth when challenged) in murine tumor models (Bramson, Graham and Gauldie, 1995; Dessureault, Graham and Gallinger, 1996; Bramson et al., 1996; Caruso et al., 1996; Xu, et al., 1996). Another ex-vivo application of recombinant adenoviral vectors expressing toxin genes such as *Pseudomonas* exotoxin and *p53* is to kill contaminating tumor cells in bone marrow harvests prior to bone marrow transplantation (Seth et al., 1996).

Adeno-associated viral vectors

Genome structure

Adeno-associated viruses (AAV) are small DNA viruses that belong to the Parvoviridae family (Berns, 1996). For productive virus replication, AAV needs a helper virus such as adenovirus or herpesvirus. However, in the absence of a helper virus, wild-type AAV can integrate into the host cell genome, thus making it an attractive vector for gene therapy (McKeon and Samulski, 1996). The AAV genome is a linear, single-stranded DNA of 4680 bp. The left half of the genome is called *rep* and encodes the four proteins that mediate replication and integration, Rep 78, 68, 52 and 40. The right half of the genome is termed *cap* and codes for the three capsid proteins VP1, VP2 and VP3. The genome is flanked by two ITR palindrome sequences of 145 bp, at both the 5' and 3' ends. ITRs are a critical component of AAV replication; they adopt a hairpin conformation that is used as the primer strand for DNA polymerase and the origin of viral replication. Other viral regulatory elements include two promoters, p5 and p19, which drive *rep* transcripts, and the p40 promoter which provides polyadenylation signals near the right end of the genome and controls coat protein transcription (Berns, 1996).

Life cycle of adeno-associated viral vectors

AAV has been shown to infect a variety of cells including epithelial cells, fibroblasts and hematopoietic cells (Berns, 1996). It has been suggested that AAV enters the cells by the process of receptor-mediated endocytosis. While the exact receptor for AAV is not yet identified, competition assays have led to the suggestion that a 150 kDa glycoprotein participates in the entry of AAV into cells (Mizukami, Young and Brown, 1996). After cell penetration, the virus enters the endocytic vesicles and is uncoated. The fate of the AAV genome in the cells depends upon the presence or absence of the helper viruses during the infection. In the absence of the helper virus, there is limited expression of the AAV regulatory proteins. Because of this, any further DNA replication is inhibited and the AAV integrates into the host genome and induces a latent infection. Wild-type AAV has been shown to integrate at a specific site on the q arm of human chromosome 19 (Samulski et al., 1991). If the AAV infection occurs in the presence of helper virus such as adenovirus or herpes virus, AAV will undergo a productive infection. Interestingly, if the cell's stress response genes are expressed, due to exposure to genotoxic agents such as γ-radiation or ultraviolet (u.v.) light, AAV genes can also be expressed, resulting in the virus replication in the absence of helper virus (Berns, 1996).

Generation of recombinant adeno-associated viruses

The overall approach to the generation of recombinant AAV vectors involves the use of two cloning vectors. One is the vector plasmid (e.g., psub201+) which carries the cDNA of interest inserted between the two AAV ITRs. The second plasmid is the helper plasmid (AAV/Ad), which does not contain any sequences homologous to the vector plasmid, but supplies the required AAV coding sequences, *cap* and *rep*, in *trans*. The two plasmids are cotransfected in a permissive cell line (generally 293 cells), and concomitantly infected with recombinant AAV (Figure 3.4). The complementation between the two vectors allows the production of recombinant AAV. The helper Rep proteins allow plasmid replication, the cap proteins lead to encapsulation and formation of infectious recombinant AAV particles, and the packaging proteins are provided by wild-type adenovirus (McCarty and Samulski, 1996; Carter and Flotte, 1996).

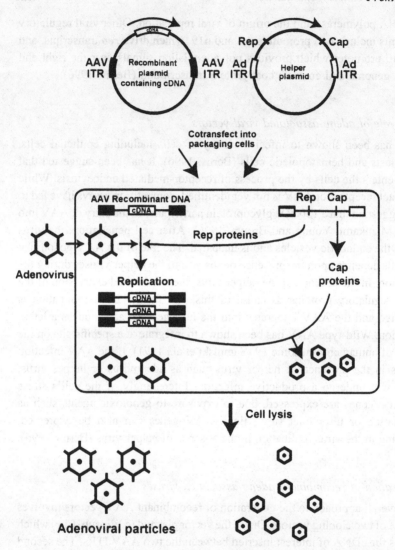

Recombinant AAV Particles

Fig. 3.4. *Construction of recombinant AAV vectors.* A recombinant AAV plasmid containing the cDNA of interest and a helper plasmid containing AAV genome are cotransfected into a producer cell line (generally 293 cells). Cells are simultaneously infected with a helper adenovirus. Helper plasmid-mediated Rep protein synthesis helps in maintaining the recombinant AAV replication, and Cap proteins produce the capsid proteins required for the recombinant AAV encapsulation. Adenovirus provides the necessary replication and packaging functions. Producer cells produce both recombinant AAV and wild-type adenovirus. Adenovirus can be heat inactivated, and recombinant AAV purified by CsCl$_2$ gradient.

Features of recombinant adeno-associated viral vectors, and recent improvements in vector development

Like retroviruses, AAV can integrate into the host chromosome. However, it is controversial as to whether the recombinant AAV used for gene therapy also integrate on chromosome 19 to any significant degree (Kearns et al., 1996). Recombinant AAV vectors are also capable of integrating the provirus into the DNA of nonmitotic cells. Thus, it is likely that recombinant AAV will find application in gene transfer into hematopoietic cells, especially stem cells. Recombinant AAV are expected to be safer than other viral vectors, since so far no disease has been associated with AAV. If AAV recombinants do integrate into cellular DNA, however, the potential risks of modifying the expression of cellular genes described with retroviruses must be considered. This risk would be minimal if integration were limited to 19q as for wild-type AAV. Recombinant AAV appear to infect several types of cells, hence the lack of cell and tissue specificity. Recombinant AAV have been constructed using tissue-specific promoters and are being tested (Doll et al., 1996; Peel et al., 1997).

Contamination with wild-type AAV and adenovirus in AAV stocks is sometimes a problem. However, new vector systems and packaging cell lines have been designed to circumvent these problems. The AAV genome in these modified vectors is flanked by adenoviral terminal repeats. This minimizes the mobilization of the helper genome and wild-type AAV contamination (Trempe, 1996). Another limitation of the commonly used method of recombinant AAV generation is that it results in cell lysis and death due to adenovirus and AAV replication, and only limited numbers of recombinant AAV virions are generated, yielding low virus titer. To circumvent this, packaging cell lines have been developed that contain either the integrated AAV genome devoid of terminal repeat sequences or adenoviral early genes or Rep genes (Holscher et al., 1994; McKeon and Samulski, 1996; Wang, Ponnazhagan and Srivastava, 1996). Using these packaging cell lines, viral stocks of as high as 10^{12} pfus/ml have been reported. Finally, AAV vectors suffer from a limitation of the size of the transgene (4.9 kb) that can be inserted.

Preclinical evaluation of recombinant adeno-associated viral vectors

In most of the initial applications of recombinant AAV, hematopoietic cells were used as the targets (McCarty and Samulski, 1996). Recently, reports have also appeared on the use of AAV vectors to express cytotoxic genes such as *p53* to kill cancer cells (Qazilbash et al., 1997); and GM-CSF, B7.1 or IL-12 for modulating the immune system (Luo et al., 1995; Doll et al.,

1996; Anderson et al., 1997; Clary et al., 1997). In all of these reports, the expression of foreign transgene in the target cells was demonstrated. AAV expressing the *MDR* gene has been shown to confer drug resistance to bone marrow cells (Baudard et al., 1996). In preclinical animal models, recombinant AAV vectors have been found to be fairly safe (Conrad et al., 1996). However, the field is still in its infancy, and it is too early to reach any clear conclusion with respect to in-vivo applications of AAV vectors for cancer gene therapy.

Other viral vectors

Pox viruses

These comprise a large family of complex DNA viruses that replicate in the cytoplasm. Their genome size varies from 130 to about 300 kbp. There are two ITR at the ends of a large genome that encodes for at least 30 proteins. Viruses enter the cell by fusing with the plasma membrane. After entry into the cytosol, DNA replicates and virions are assembled and released from the cells (Moss, 1991). Foreign DNA can be inserted into the pox genome by the process of homologous recombination or by in-vitro ligation. Several features of pox viruses have led to their extensive use as expression vectors (Moss, 1991). These features include the ease with which recombinant vectors can be formed and isolated; the large capacity of pox viruses for foreign DNA; the relatively high level of transgene expression; and the wide host range. Although pox virus promoters can drive gene expression, other cognate promoters can also be used. Recombinant pox viral vectors (vaccinia, fowl pox, canary pox) have been extensively used for expressing the heterologous proteins such as cytokines, CEA antigens, prostate-specific antigen (PSA) for vaccination purposes, and antigens for immunotherapeutic purposes (Hodge et al., 1994, 1995; Paoletti, 1996; Lattime et al., 1996; Ratliff et al., 1996; Moss et al., 1996). In one report, a recombinant pox virus expressing p53 protein protected mice from a challenge with isogenic and highly immuno-genic murine fibroblast tumor cells expressing a mutant human p53 but lacking murine p53 (Roth et al., 1996). Two clinical trial using a vaccinia vector expressing CEA and PSA antigens have been initiated.

Herpes simplex viruses

These viruses belong to the family Herpesviridae and include herpes simplex types 1 and 2 (HSV-1 and HSV-2). The viral vectors have been primarily developed for targeting the central nervous system (Glorioso, DeLucca and

Fink, 1995). Much of the published work has been done using HSV-1 based vectors. HSV-1 can either undergo productive infection, and express lytic function, or the virus may express latency genes and stay in the latent state without undergoing viral replication. HSV-1 is a large, enveloped virus that has a double-stranded DNA of about 150 kb long. The genome is split into a long (U_L) and a short (U_S) segment, both of which are flanked by ITR. For the viral lytic cycle to take place, several regulatory proteins must be expressed, including immediate early (IE), early (E) and late (L) viral genes. For gene therapy purposes, it is possible to design HSV vectors that minimize the viral replication. Recombinant HSV-1 can be constructed by replacing the immediate early gene, *IE3* gene, with the cDNA of interest, and the virus can be rescued in a packaging cell line that provides the *IE3* gene product (ICP4 protein) in *trans* (Johnson and Friedmann, 1994; Marconi et al., 1996). The use of plasmid-based 'amplicons' has also been proposed instead of whole virus-based vectors (Ho, 1994).

Features of HSV vectors include their ability to be grown to high titers (10^{11}–10^{12} pfus/ml); their ability to infect nondividing cells; and their ability to package large inserts. Problems associated with the use of HSV vectors are the difficulty in completely eliminating lytic viral gene expression and therefore cytotoxicity, and the transient nature of gene expression. Despite these problems, several genes have been expressed successfully by HSV vectors. These include hepatitis B surface antigens, alpha interferon, and hypoxanthine phosphoribosyl transferase (Glorioso et al., 1995; Fink and Glorioso, 1997). The marker genes *lacZ*, nerve growth factor and human *NGFp75* have been expressed from amplicons (Glorioso et al., 1995). So far, there have been no clinical protocols utilizing the HSV-based vectors.

HIV *vectors*

Although initially proposed for their application to anti-HIV gene therapy, HIV-based vectors (a subclass of retroviruses termed lentiviruses) are worthy of exploring for cancer gene therapy because they can be targeted to CD4+ cells, and can deliver to dividing as well as to nondividing cells (Poeschla, Corbeau and Wong-Staal, 1996). Like MoMuLV, HIV-1 genome also has *gag, pol* and *env* genes and 5'- and 3'-LTR. However, the genome also contains six additional genes – *tat, rev, nef, vif, vpr*, and *vpu*. To generate recombinant HIV-1 vectors, the 5'-LTR is linked with a 5' leader sequence comprising a portion of the *gag* gene, the *rev* response elements, a marker gene (such as *neo*[R]) and the 3'-LTR. Virus can be packaged in the producer cell lines after doubly selecting for stable expression of viral proteins (Naldini et al., 1996).

The presence of a nuclear targeting signal in the accessory protein Vpr permits the integration of the genome into the cell nuclei even in nondividing cells (Poeschla et al., 1996). Like MoMuLV retroviruses, HIV-based vectors have also been constructed using VSV G protein pseudotyping to increase the host range. Although in-vitro gene transfer of many marker genes by the lenti vectors has been demonstrated, their in-vivo applications, particularly in the clinic, remain to be studied. Their ability to transduce nondividing cells, which is not the case for other retroviruses, makes them attractive for some types of gene therapy.

Hybrid vectors

To exploit the best properties of two vectors, hybrid vectors have been produced in recent years. One such vector is a hybrid between adenovirus and AAV (Fisher et al., 1996b). For the construction of this virus, a proviral clone of the AAV genome was inserted in place of E1 using the methodology developed for constructing recombinant adenoviruses. A *rep* expression plasmid was conjugated with the hybrid virus through a polylysine linker. In theory, this virus will deliver recombinant AAV genomes using adenovirus as a shuttle vector. Another hybrid vector that incorporates critical elements of HSV-1 amplicon vectors and AAV vectors has also been constructed (Johnston et al., 1997). The hybrid vector contains the HSV-1 origin of DNA replication, OriS, and the DNA cleavage/packaging signal *pac*, which allow amplicon replication and packaging in HSV-1 virions. This vector permits expression of transgene under the control of its own promoter, but the latter is flanked by AAV ITR sequences such that it can be integrated. Thus, this vector combines the best features of HSV-1, such as cell infectability and capacity to package large genomic sequences, with the ability of AAV to integrate into chromosomes. Such vectors have been shown to allow long-term gene expression in both dividing and nondividing cells (Johnston et al., 1997). Other types of hybrid vectors described in the literature include pseudo-retroviruses, discussed in the previous section.

Replicating viral vectors

While most of our efforts in gene therapy have been directed towards developing replication-deficient viral vectors, some interesting approaches in the development of viral vectors that undergo replication only in tumor cells but not in normal cells have recently been proposed. One such vector is an adenovirus deletion mutant, dl1520 (Bischoff et al., 1996). This mutant lacks a 55 kDa protein encoded by the E1b gene of adenovirus. The function of this protein in the wild-type adenovirus is to bind to the tumor suppressor gene *p53*, and hence inactivate its ability to block cell cycle progression. This is because cell division is needed for viral DNA replication to proceed. The adenovirus mutant lacking E1b-expressing 55 kDa protein cannot replicate in cells that express a normal endogenous p53 protein, because the ability of *p53* to induce growth arrest remains unchecked. However, this vector will replicate in cells that have defective p53 functions. It has been shown that dl1520 virus kills tumor cells that express a mutant *p53* or that are null for *p53* much more effectively than cells that express wild-type *p53* (Bischoff et al., 1996). This vector has also been shown to be capable of inhibiting the growth of human xenografts (expressing defective *p53*) in nude mice. Currently, this virus is being tested in a Phase I clinical trial. Similarly, papilloma virus mutants defective in E6 or E7 functions cannot inactivate p53 (E6 deletion) and Rb (E7 deletion) proteins. Therefore, these vectors should also replicate in tumor cells defective in p53 and Rb functions, respectively.

Similarly, HSV-1 mutant lacking ribonucleotide reductase and thymidine kinase enzymes can preferentially grow in dividing but not in nondividing cells because these two HSV-1 encoded enzymes are essential for viral DNA synthesis in quiescent cells, whereas in actively dividing cells these enzymes are not essential. Since HSV-1-based vectors might induce neurotoxicity, the gene responsible for such negative effects, *ICP-34.5*, has been further mutated (Kucharczuk et al., 1997). Another virus that replicates mainly in transformed cells is minute virus of mice, an autonomously replicating parvovirus (Corsini et al., 1996). Since many applications of viral vectors in vivo involve local administration into the tumor site, the use of such replication competent vectors could clearly have a benefit in spreading the effects of the vector across the whole tumor mass.

Epstein–Barr virus

Epstein–Barr virus (EBV) vectors belong to the herpes virus family, and have the unique capacity of being able to replicate extrachromosomally in the cell nuclei (Mucke et al., 1997). EBV accomplishes this by utilizing a cis-acting origin of replication OriP, and a transactivating gene product EBNA-1, which activates the OriP. Under the control of cellular genes, EBV episomes are replicated once per cell cycle. EBV-based vectors containing OriP and EBNA-1 can be constructed in appropriate bacterial plasmids, and the foreign gene of interest can be cloned into this vector for delivery into the nuclei. EBV vectors dependent upon the expression of EBNA-1 have also been designed to cause lysis of tumor cells infected with EBV but not of normal cells (Judde et al., 1996).

Nonviral vectors

DNA of choice can be also delivered to the cell nucleus by using nonviral methods, the simplest of which is the use of plasmid DNA expression vectors driven by eukaryotic promoters. Such plasmids can be injected directly into the tissue or tumor of choice (Wolff et al., 1990). Although this a simple approach, the efficiency of gene delivery is poor. To increase the transfection efficiency, many physicochemical methods have been devised and are discussed below.

Liposomes

To increase the DNA delivery to cells, plasmid DNA can be used in combination with liposomes. Since DNA is negatively charged, it can form complexes with positively charged liposomes. The utility of various types of liposomes has been explored, including that of monocationic liposomes such as lipofectin, which is a mixture of DOTMA and DOPE, polycationic liposomes, and cationic derivatives of cholesterol and diacyl glycerol (Felgner et al., 1995; Bedu-Addo et al., 1996). DNA can also be trapped inside the aqueous interior of the liposomes, in which case negatively charged pH-sensitive liposomes whose membranes are destablized at low pH can also be used (Legendre and Szoka, 1992). Liposomal-mediated DNA delivery methods are routinely used for in-vitro transfections. These methods have also been employed in vivo in animal tumor models to express *p53*, suicide genes for inducing cytotoxicity, antisense to the *ras* oncogene, cytokine genes, *HLA-B7* to activate immune cells, and *MDR* for chemoprotection (Yagi et al., 1994; Nabel et al., 1996; Aksentijevich et al., 1996; Hsiao et al., 1997). Many clinical protocols employing liposome-mediated gene therapy especially for vaccine purposes (using genes such as *HLA-B7*) are being actively pursued (Nabel et al., 1996).

Particle bombardment

DNA entry into cells can be accomplished by physical means such as particle bombardment, commonly referred to as the gene gun method. In this technique, the DNA of choice is coated onto microscopic particles (generally gold particles) that are accelerated by a motive force to a velocity sufficient to cause them to penetrate cells. The physical force can be generated by a high-voltage electric discharge, a helium pressure discharge, or by other means (Johnston and Tang, 1994). Using this gene gun-mediated approach, the transfer of several genes, including marker genes, growth hormones, and alpha antitrypsin, has been accomplished in vitro (Yang and Sun, 1995; Qiu et al., 1996). The gene gun approach has also been used for gene transfer purposes in vivo, mainly for immunotherapy purposes using plasmids encoding for IL-6, IL-12, and hemaglutin antigen, which are injected into various organ sites (intramuscular, intratumoral, skin) in murine models. In these experiments, strong cytotoxic T lymphocyte responses against the tumor cells, which result in tumor regression, have been reported (Pertmer et al., 1995; Sun et al., 1995; Rakhmilevich et al., 1996; Feltquate et al., 1997; Torres et al., 1997).

Receptor-mediated endocytosis

It has also been shown that plasmid DNA can be delivered via receptor-mediated endocytosis. With this technique, the route of DNA delivery can be controlled by using specific ligands conjugated to the plasmid DNAs. Various ligands such as asialoglycoprotein, transferin, folate, mannose receptor, and CD3 antigen have been used (Plank et al., 1992; Buschle et al., 1995; Cheng, 1996). Liposomes have been used in addition to DNAs conjugated to these ligands in some studies (Koike et al., 1994; Kikuchi et al., 1996; Lee and Huang, 1996). Much of this work has been done in-vitro using various cell lines, but these approaches are being tested in in-vivo models.

Features of nonviral-based vectors

The advantage of using plasmid DNAs – alone or in combination with other approaches discussed above – for gene therapy is the minimum level of toxicity caused by these vectors to the host. Moreover, all plasmid-based vectors can deliver DNA to a greater or lesser extent to most target cells in vitro. Plasmid DNAs have no tissue specificity, but they are relatively easily modified for targeting purposes, e.g., for transcriptional targeting or tissue-specific targeting.

The main limitation of plasmid-based gene therapy is the relatively low levels of gene transfer, and short expression times. Most of the DNA delivered to the cells remains trapped in membrane-limited vesicles and is degraded in lysosomes. To overcome this problem, attempts to push the trapped DNA out of the endosomes have been made by using plasmid DNA in combination with adenoviruses. Work in our laboratory has shown that during internalization of adenovirus into the cell, the adenovirus disrupts the endosome membrane to escape into the cytosol (see Figure 3.2). Interestingly, if other molecules such as DNA are co-internalized with adenovirus into the endosome, adenovirus also increases the transfection efficiency of such DNAs into the cells by avoiding lysosomal degradation. Monocationic and polycationic liposomes can further increase such viral-mediated transfection (Yoshimura et al., 1993; Seth et al., 1994; P. Seth, unpublished data). Interestingly, u.v.-inactivated adenovirus or empty capsids (i.e., devoid of any DNA) also mediated the plasmid transfection, indicating that adenoviral genome is not required for adenoviral-mediated DNA uptake into the cell nucleus (Seth et al., 1994; Seth, 1994b). Using these methods, we have delivered a variety of DNAs (> 40 kb), including some of the toxin genes (such as *Pseudomonas* exotoxin) into the cells (Seth et al., 1996). Moreover, by linking plasmid DNA and/or adenovirus with other ligands such as epidermal growth factor, or transferrin, DNA can be delivered into cells through specific receptors (Seth, 1994c; De et al., in press). Adenoviruses can be also used in combination with other receptor-mediated DNA delivery methods described above (Michael et al., 1993; Fisher and Wilson, 1994; Schwarzenberger et al., 1996). These combination methods, though not yet tried in a clinical setting, deserve further attention.

Conclusions and future directions for improving vector-based cancer gene therapy

Since the idea of vector-based gene therapy was originally proposed, a great deal of progress in vector development has been made. It is clear that the existing vectors have provided excellent tools to learn the basic science of gene therapy, and will find some application in cancer gene therapy. They have proved to be capable of effectively targeting and delivering genes in vitro, and have shown limited success in in-vivo gene delivery in animal models. Particularly important, in Phase I clinical trials, most of the vectors have been found to be safe.

Although it may be too early for a final judgment, it is probable that none of the current vectors will be adequate for cancer gene therapy (Verma, 1994; Vile, 1996). Given the fact that human cancer spreads systemically, the evolution of gene therapy approaches into curative cancer treatment is likely to be an uphill task. Although the local delivery of the vectors, e.g., for treating residual disease, and for other in-vitro and ex-vivo purposes (as discussed in various chapters in this book), should be maximally exploited, the ultimate success of cancer gene therapy depends upon the induction of a vector-mediated systemic effect. Perhaps we need to combine several vector-mediated cancer gene therapy approaches, for example the use of an enzyme/prodrug system, combined in the same vector, with components designed to induce immunomodulation. One can also use multiple vectors in a single regimen. It seems possible that cancer gene therapy in combination with other conventional cancer treatment approaches could also be potentially useful.

In general, the in-vivo transduction efficacy of most vectors is too low to be effective in cancer gene therapy. Vectors that induce a bystander effect, or replication-restricted vectors, can at least in part overcome this problem, and hence research in this area is likely to be valuable. Novel vectors that can target both the dividing and nondividing cells should also be further explored, and methods will need to be developed whereby vectors are modified in such a way that multiple administrations (if needed) will be feasible.

Another area where research is much needed is in the development of vectors in which the expression of the transgene is efficiently controlled, at least in those approaches to cancer gene therapy which rely on long-term continuous expression of the protein. The use of tissue-specific regulatory elements to drive the transgene expression is also worthy of greater research efforts. Although some progress has been made in this direction in recent years, much of the work so far has been conducted using the promoters and enhancers already present in the viral genome. Unfortunately, these are very often shut off by the host. The possibility of incorporating regulatory elements that lead to repression of transgene transcription in specific types of normal cells should also be considered. Ideally, vectors should have a built-in mechanism that permits them to target cancer cells and not to enter the normal cells in the body even where tumor-specific promoters are used, since this would permit the administration of lower viral titers and lessen the risk of toxicities. It would also overcome the potential harmful effects that overexpression of transgene could produce in the patient.

Before specific vectors are taken to Phase I clinical trials, we must provide evidence that the concept on which they are based is valid, using in-vitro, in-vivo and ex-vivo assays (whichever is applicable). Better in-vivo assays will require the development of more appropriate animal models. It will be essential for basic scientists to work in close association with clinical scientists, not only in developing novel vectors but also in designing, executing, and evaluating the results of clinical trials. In brief, cancer gene therapy, like most conventional forms of cancer therapy, will have to be conducted by teams, but teams that include new members – basic scientists!

References

Aksentijevich, I., Pastan, I., Lunardi-Iskandar, Y., Gallo, R. C., Gottesman, M. M. and Thierry, A. R. (1996). In vitro and in vivo liposome-mediated gene transfer leads to human MDR1 expression in mouse bone marrow progenitor cells. *Human Gene Therapy*, **7**: 1111–22.

Anderson, R., MacDonald, I., Corbett, T., Hacking, G., Lowdell, M. W. and Prentice, H. G. (1997). Construction and biological characterization of an interleukin-12 fusion protein (Flexi-12): delivery to acute myeloid leukemic blasts using adeno-associated virus. *Human Gene Therapy*. **8**: 1125–35.

Armentano, D., Sookdeo, C. C., Hehir, K. M., Gregory, R. J., St George, J. A., Prince, G. A., Wadsworth, S. C. and Smith, A. E. (1995). Characterization of an adenovirus gene transfer vector containing an E4 deletion. *Human Gene Therapy*, **6**: 1343–53.

Battini, J. L., Heard, J. M. and Danos, O. (1992). Receptor choice determinants in the envelope glycoproteins of amphotropic, xenotropic, and polytropic murine leukemia viruses. *Journal of Virology*, **66**: 1468–75.

Baudard, M., Flotte, T. R., Aran, J. M., Thierry, A. R., Pastan, I., Pang, M. G., Kearns, W. G. and Gottesman, M. M. (1996). Expression of the human multidrug resistance and glucocerebrosidase cDNAs from adeno-associated vectors: efficient promoter activity of AAV sequences and in vivo delivery via liposomes. *Human Gene Therapy*, **7**: 1309–22.

Bedu-Addo, F. K., Tang, P., Xu, Y. and Huang, L. (1996). Interaction of poly-ethyleneglycol–phospholipid conjugates with cholesterol–phosphatidylcholine mixtures: sterically stabilized liposome formulations. *Pharmacology Research*, **13**: 718–24.

Bender, M. A., Palmer, T. D., Gelinas, R. E. and Miller, A. D. (1987). Evidence that the packaging signal of Moloney murine leukemia virus extends into the gag region. *Journal of Virology*, **61**: 1639–46.

Bergelson, J. M., Cunningham, J. A., Droguett, G., Kurt-Jones, E. A., Krithivas, A., Hong, J. S., Horwitz, M. S., Crowell, R. L. and Finberg, R. W. (1997). Isolation of a common receptor for Coxsackie B viruses and adenoviruses 2 and 5. *Science*, **275**: 1320–3.

Berns, K. L. (1996). Parvoviridae: The viruses and their replication. In B. N. Fields, D. M. Knippe and P. Howley (eds.) *Fields Virology*, pp. 2173–97. Lippincott-Raven, Philadelphia.

Bett, A. J., Haddara, W., Prevec, L. and Graham, F. L. (1994). An efficient and flexible system for construction of adenovirus vectors with insertions or deletions in early regions 1 and 3. *Proceedings of the National Academy of Sciences of the United States of America*, **91**: 8802–06.

Bischoff, J. R., Kirn, D. H., Williams, A., Heise, C., Horn, S., Muna, M., Ng, L., Nye, J. A., Sampson-Johannes, A., Fattaey, A. and McCormick, F. (1996). An adenovirus mutant that replicates selectively in p53-deficient human tumor cells. *Science*, **274**: 373–6.

Bramson, J. L., Graham, F. L. and Gauldie, J. (1995). The use of adenoviral vectors for gene therapy and gene transfer in vivo. *Current Opinion in Biotechnology*, **6**: 590–5.

Bramson, J. L., Hitt, M., Addison, C. L., Muller, W. J., Gauldie, J. and Graham, F. L. (1996). Direct intratumoral injection of an adenovirus expressing interleukin-12 induces regression and long-lasting immunity that is associated with highly localized expression of interleukin-12. *Human Gene Therapy*, 7: 1995–2002.

Bunnell, B. A., Metzger, M., Byrne, E., Morgan, R. A. and Donahue, R. E. (1997). Efficient in vivo marking of primary CD4+ T lymphocytes in nonhuman primates using a gibbon ape leukemia virus-derived retroviral vector. *Blood*, **89**: 1987–95.

Buschle, M., Cotten, M., Kirlappos, H., Mechtler, K., Schaffner, G., Zauner, W., Birnstiel, M. L. and Wagner, E. (1995). Receptor-mediated gene transfer into human T lymphocytes via binding of DNA/CD3 antibody particles to the CD3 T cell receptor complex. *Human Gene Therapy*, **6**: 753–61.

Cai, D. W., Mukhopadhyay, T., Liu, Y., Fujiwara, T. and Roth, J. A. (1993). Stable expression of the wild-type p53 gene in human lung cancer cells after retrovirus-mediated gene transfer. *Human Gene Therapy*, **4**: 617–24.

Carter, B. J. and Flotte, T. R. (1996). Development of adeno-associated virus vectors for gene therapy of cystic fibrosis. *Current Topics in Microbiology and Immunology*, **218**: 119–44.

Caruso, M., Pham-Nguyen, K., Kwong, Y. L., Xu, B., Kosai, K. I., Finegold, M., Woo, S. L. and Chen, S. H. (1996). Adenovirus-mediated interleukin-12 gene therapy for metastatic colon carcinoma. *Proceedings of the National Academy of Sciences of the United States of America*, **93**: 11302–06.

Cheng, P. W. (1996). Receptor ligand-facilitated gene transfer: enhancement of liposome-mediated gene transfer and expression by transferrin. *Human Gene Therapy*, **7**: 275–82.

Clary, B. M., Coveney, E. C., Blazer, D. G. 3rd, Philip, R., Philip, M., Morse, M., Gilboa, E. and Lyerly, H. K. (1997). Active immunization with tumor cells transduced by a novel AAV plasmid-based gene delivery system. *Journal of Immunotherapy*, **20**: 26–37.

Coffin, J. M. (1996). Retroviridae: The viruses and their replication. In B. N. Fields, D. M. Knippe and P. Howley (eds.) *Fields Virology*, pp. 1767–840. Lippincott-Raven, Philadelphia.

Cone, R. D. and Mulligan, R. C. (1992). High-efficiency gene transfer into mammalian cells: generation of helper-free recombinant retrovirus with broad mammalian host range. *Biotechnology*, **24**: 420–4.

Conrad, C. K., Allen, S. S., Afione, S. A., Reynolds, T. C., Beck, S. E., Fee-Maki, M., Barrazza-Ortiz, X., Adams, R., Askin, F. B. and Carter, B. J. (1996). Safety of single-dose administration of an adeno-associated virus (AAV)-CFTR vector in the primate lung. *Gene Therapy*, **3**: 658–68.

Corsini, J., Afanasiev, B., Maxwell, I. H. and Carlson, J. O. (1996). Autonomous parvovirus and densovirus gene vectors. *Advances in Virus Research*, **47**: 303–51.

Cosset, F. L. and Russell, S. J. (1996). Targeting retrovirus entry. *Gene Therapy*, **3**: 946–56.

Craig, C., Wersto, R., Kim, M., Ohri, E., Li, Z., Katayose, D., Lee, S. J., Trepel, J., Cowan, K. and Seth, P. A. (1997). A recombinant adenovirus expressing p27[Kip1] induces cell cycle arrest and loss of cyclin-Cdk activity in human breast cancer cells. *Oncogene*, **14**: 2283–9.

Dai, Y., Schwarz, E. M., Gu, D., Zhang, W. W., Sarvetnick, N. and Verma, I. M. (1995). Cellular and humoral immune responses to adenoviral vectors containing factor IX gene: tolerization of factor IX and vector antigens allows for long-term expression. *Proceedings of the National Academy of Sciences of the United States of America*, **92**: 1401–05.

Danos, O. and Mulligan, R. C. (1988). Safe and efficient generation of recombinant retroviruses with amphotropic and ecotropic host ranges. *Proceedings of* the National Academy of Sciences of the United States of America, **85**: 6460–4.

De, S. K., Venkatetshan, C. N. S., Seth, P., Gajdusek, D. C. and Gibbs, C. J. (1998). Adenovirus-mediated human immunodeficiency virus-1 Nef expression in human monocytes/macrophages and effect of Nef on downmodulation of Fcγ receptors and expression on monokines. *Blood*, **91**: (in press).

Deryckere, F. and Burgert, H. G. (1996). Tumor necrosis factor alpha induces the adenovirus early 3 promoter by activation of NF-kappaB. *Journal of Biological Chemistry*, **271**: 30249–55.

Dessureault, S., Graham, F. and Gallinger, S. (1996). B7-1 gene transfer into human cancer cells by infection with an adenovirus-B7 (Ad-B7) expression vector. *Annals of Surgical Oncology*, **3**: 317–24.

Dilloo, D., Rill, D. R., Grossmann, M. E., Leimig, T. and Brenner, M. K. (1996). Gene marking and gene therapy for transplantation medicine. *Journal of Hematotherapy*, **5**: 553–5.

Doll, R. F., Crandall, J. E., Dyer, C. A., Aucoin, J. M. and Smith, F. I. (1996). Comparison of promoter strengths on gene delivery into mammalian brain cells using AAV vectors. *Gene Therapy*, **3**: 437–47.

Donahue, R. E., Kessler, S. W., Bodine, D. et al. (1992). Helper virus induced T cell lymphoma in nonhuman primates after retroviral mediated gene transfer. *Journal of Experimental Medicine*, **176**: 1125–35.

Dong, Y., Wen, P., Manome, Y., Parr, M., Hirshowitz, A., Chen, L., Hirschowitz, E. A., Crystal, R., Weichselbaum, R., Kufe, D. W. and Fine, H. A. (1996). In vivo replication-deficient adenovirus vector-mediated transduction of the cytosine deaminase gene sensitizes glioma cells to 5-fluorocytosine. *Human Gene Therapy*, **7**: 713–20.

Dranoff, G., Jaffee, E., Lazenby, A., Golumbek, P., Levitsky, H., Brose, K., Jackson, V., Hamada, H., Pardoll, D. and Mulligan, R. C. (1993). Vaccination with irradiated tumor cells engineered to secrete murine granulocyte–macrophage colony-stimulating factor stimulates potent, specific, and long-lasting anti-tumor immunity. *Proceedings of the National Academy of Sciences of the United States of America*, **90**, 3539–43.

Elshami, A. A., Saavedra, A., Zhang, H., Kucharczuk, J. C., Spray, D. C., Fishman, G. I., Amin, K. M., Kaiser, L. R. and Albelda, S. M. (1996). Gap junctions play a role in the 'bystander effect' of the herpes simplex virus thymidine kinase/ ganciclovir system in vitro. *Gene Therapy*, **3**: 85–92.

Engelhardt, J. F., Litzky, L. and Wilson, J. M. (1994). Prolonged transgene expression in cotton rat lung with recombinant adenoviruses defective in E2a. *Human Gene Therapy*, **5**: 1217–29.

Felgner, P. L., Tsai, Y. J., Sukhu, L., Wheeler, C. J., Manthorpe, M., Marshall, J. and Cheng, S. H. (1995). Improved cationic lipid formulations for in vivo gene therapy. *Annals of the New York Academy of Sciences*, **772**: 126–39.

Feltquate, D. M., Heaney, S., Webster, R. G. and Robinson, H. L. (1997). Different T helper cell types and antibody isotypes generated by saline and gene gun DNA immunization. *Journal of Immunology*, **158**: 2278–84.

Feng, M., Cabrera, G., Deshane, J., Scanlon, K. J. and Curiel, D. T. (1995). Neoplastic reversion accomplished by high efficiency adenoviral-mediated delivery of an anti-ras ribozyme. *Cancer Research*, **55**: 2024–8.

Fink, D. J. and Glorioso, J. C. (1997). Herpes simplex virus-based vectors: problems and some solutions. *Advances in Neurology*, **72**: 149–56.

Fisher, K. J. and Wilson, J. M. (1994). Biochemical and functional analysis of an adenovirus-based ligand complex for gene transfer. *Biochemical Journal*, **299**: 49–58.

Fisher, K. J., Choi, H., Burda, J., Chen, S. J. and Wilson, J. M. (1996a). Recombinant adenovirus deleted of all viral genes for gene therapy of cystic fibrosis. *Virology*, **217**: 11–22.

Fisher, K. J., Kelley, W. M., Burda, J. F. and Wilson, J. M. (1996b). A novel adenovirus–adeno-associated virus hybrid vector that displays efficient rescue and delivery of the AAV genome. *Human Gene Therapy*, **7**: 2079–87.

Glorioso, J. C., DeLuca, N. A. and Fink, D. J. (1995). Development and application of herpes simplex virus vectors for human gene therapy. *Annual Review of Microbiology*, **49**: 675–710.

Griscelli, F., Opolon, P., Chianale, C., Di Falco, N., Franz, W. M., Perricaudet, M. and Ragot, T. (1997). Expression from cardiomyocyte-specific promoter after adenovirus-mediated gene transfer in vitro and in vivo. *CR Academic Sciences III*, **320**: 103–12.

Gunzburg, W. H. and Salmons, B. (1996). Development of retroviral vectors as safe, targeted gene delivery systems. *Journal of Molecular Medicine*, **74**: 171–82.

Guo, Z. S., Wang, L. H., Eisensmith, R. C. and Woo, S. L. (1996). Evaluation of promoter strength for hepatic gene expression in vivo following adenovirus-mediated gene transfer. *Gene Therapy*, **3**: 802–10.

Hardy, S., Kitamura, M., Harris-Stansil, T., Dai, Y. and Phipps, M. L. (1997). Construction of adenovirus vectors through Cre-lox recombination. *Journal of Virology*, **71**: 1842–9.

Ho, D. Y. (1994). Amplicon-based herpes simplex virus vectors. *Methods in Cell Biology*, **43**: 191–210.

Hoatlin, M. E., Kozak, S. L., Spiro, C. and Kabat, D. (1995). Amplified and tissue-directed expression of retroviral vectors using ping-pong techniques. *Journal of Molecular Medicine*, **73**: 113–20.

Hodge, J. W., Abrams, S., Schlom, J. and Kantor, J. A. (1994). Induction of antitumor immunity by recombinant vaccinia viruses expressing B7-1 or B7-2 costimulatory molecules. *Cancer Research*, **54**: 5552–5.

Hodge, J. W., Schlom, J., Donohue, S. J., Tomaszewski, J. E., Wheeler, C. W., Levine, B. S., Gritz, L. and Kantor, J. A. (1995). A recombinant vaccinia virus expressing human prostate-specific antigen (PSA): safety and immunogenicity in a non-human primate. *International Journal of Cancer*, **63**: 231–7.

Holscher, C., Horer, M., Kleinschmidt, J. A., Zentgraf, H., Burkle, A. and Heilbronn, R. (1994). Cell lines inducibly expressing the adeno-associated virus (AAV) rep gene: requirements for productive replication of rep-negative AAV mutants. *Journal of Virology*, **68**: 7169–77.

Hsiao, M., Tse, V., Carmel, J., Tsai, Y., Felgner, P. L., Haas, M. and Silverberg, G. D. (1997). Intracavitary liposome-mediated p53 gene transfers into glioblastoma with endogenous wild-type p53 in vivo results in tumor suppression and long-term survival. *Biochemical and Biophysical Research Communications*, **233**: 359–64.

Hwu, P., Shafer, G. E., Treisman, J., Schlindler, D. G., Gross, G., Cowherd, R., Rosenberg, S. A. and Eshhar, Z. (1993). Lysis of ovarian cancer cells by human lymphocytes redirected with a chimeric gene composed of an antibody variable region and the Fc receptor gamma chain. *Journal of Experimental Medicine*, **178**: 361–6.

Johnson, P. A. and Friedmann, T. (1994). Replication-defective recombinant herpes simplex virus vectors. *Methods in Cell Biology*, **43**: 211–30.

Johnston, K. M., Jacoby, D., Pechan, P. A., Fraeffl, C., Borghesani, P., Schuback, D.,

Dunn, R. J., Smith, F. I. and Breakfield, X. O. (1997). HSV/AAV hybrid amplicon vectors extend transgene expression in human glioma cells. *Human Gene Therapy*, 8: 359–70.

Johnston, S. A. and Tang, D. C. (1994). Gene gun transfection of animal cells and genetic immunization. *Methods in Cell Biology*, 43: 353–65.

Judde, J. G., Spangler, G., Magrath, I. and Bhatia, K. (1996). Use of Epstein–Barr virus nuclear antigen-1 in targeted therapy of EBV-associated neoplasia. *Human Gene Therapy*, 7: 647–53.

Kass-Eisler, A., Leinwand, L., Gall, J., Bloom, B. and Falck-Pedersen, E. (1996). Circumventing the immune response to adenovirus-mediated gene therapy. *Gene Therapy*, 3: 154–62.

Katayose, D., Gudas, J., Nguyen, H., Srivastava, S., Cowan, K. and Seth, P. (1995a). Cytotoxic effects of a recombinant adenovirus expressing human wild type p53 on tumor and normal mammary epithelial cells. *Clinical Cancer Research*, 8: 889–98.

Katayose, D., Wersto, R., Cowan, K. H. and Seth, P. (1995b). Effects of a recombinant adenovirus expressing WAF1/Cip1 on cell growth, cell cycle, and apoptosis. *Cell Growth and Differentiation*, 6: 1207–12.

Kavanaugh, M. P., Miller, D. G., Zhang, W., Law, W., Kozak, S. L., Kabat, D. and Miller, A. D. (1994). Cell-surface receptors for gibbon ape leukemia virus and amphotropic murine retrovirus are inducible sodium-dependent phosphate symporters. *Proceedings of the National Academy of Sciences of the United States of America*, 91: 7071–5.

Kearns, W. G., Afione, S. A., Fulmer, S. B., Pang, M. C., Erikson, D., Egan, M., Landrum, M. J., Flotte, T. R. and Cutting, G. R. (1996). Recombinant adeno-associated virus (AAV-CFTR) vectors do not integrate in a site-specific fashion in an immortalized epithelial cell line. *Gene Therapy*, 3: 748–55.

Kijima, H., Ishida, H., Ohkawa, T., Kashani-Sabet, M. and Scanlon, K. J. (1995). Therapeutic applications of ribozymes. *Pharmacological Therapy*, 68: 247–67.

Kikuchi, A., Sugaya, S., Ueda, H., Tanaka, K., Aramaki, Y., Hara, T., Arima, H., Tsuchiya, S. and Fuwa, T. (1996). Efficient gene transfer to EGF receptor overexpressing cancer cells by means of EGF-labeled cationic liposomes. *Biochemistry and Biophysics Research Communication*, 227: 666–71.

Koike, K., Hara, T., Aramaki, Y., Takada, S. and Tsuchiya, S. (1994). Receptor-mediated gene transfer into hepatic cells using asialoglycoprotein-labeled liposomes. *Annals of the New York Academy of Sciences*, 716: 331–3.

Krasnykh, V. N., Mikheeva, G. V., Douglas, J. T. and Curiel, D. T. (1996). Generation of recombinant adenovirus vectors with modified fibers for altering viral tropism. *Journal of Virology*, 70: 6839–46.

Kucharczuk, J. C., Randazzo, B., Chang, M. Y. et al. (1997). Use of a 'replication-restricted' herpes virus to treat experimental human malignant mesothelioma. *Cancer Research*, 57: 466–71.

Lan, K. H., Kanai, F., Shiratori, Y., Okabe, S., Yoshida, Y., Wakimoto, H., Hamada, H., Tanaka, T., Ohashi, M. and Omata, M. (1996). Tumor-specific gene expression in carcinoembryonic antigen-producing gastric cancer cells using adenovirus vectors. *Gastroenterology*, 111: 1241–51.

Lattime, E. C., Lee, S. S., Eisenlohr, L. C. and Mastrangelo, M. J. (1996). In situ cytokine gene transfection using vaccinia virus vectors. *Seminars in Oncology*, 23: 88–100.

Lee, R. J. and Huang, L. (1996). Folate-targeted, anionic liposome-entrapped polylysine-condensed DNA for tumor cell-specific gene transfer. *Journal of Biological Chemistry*, 271: 8481–7.

Legendre, J. Y. and Szoka, F. C. Jr (1992). Delivery of plasmid DNA into mammalian cell lines using pH-sensitive liposomes: comparison with cationic liposomes. *Pharmacology Research*, **9**: 1235–42.

Li, Z., Shanmugam, N., Katayose, D., Huber, B., Srivastava, S., Cowan, K. and Seth, P. (1997). Enzyme/prodrug gene therapy approach for breast cancer using a recombinant adenovirus expressing *Escherichia coli* cytosine deaminase. *Cancer Gene Therapy*, **4**: 113–17.

Licht, T., Aksentijevich, I., Gottesman, M. M. and Pastan, I. (1995). Efficient expression of functional human MDR1 gene in murine bone marrow after retroviral transduction of purified hematopoietic stem cells. *Blood*, **86**: 111–21.

Luo, F., Zhou, S. Z., Cooper, S., Munshi, N. C., Boswell, H. S., Broxmeyer, H. E. and Srivastava, A. (1995). Adeno-associated virus 2-mediated gene transfer and functional expression of the human granulocyte–macrophage colony-stimulating factor. *Experimental Hematology*, **23**: 1261–7.

Lynch, C. M. and Miller, A. D. (1991). Production of high-titer helper virus-free retroviral vectors by cocultivation of packaging cells with different host ranges. *Journal of Virology*, **65**: 3887–90.

Marconi, P., Krisky, D., Oligino, T., Poliani, P. L., Ramakrishnan, R., Goins, W. F., Fink, D. J. and Glorioso, J. C. (1996). Replication-defective herpes simplex virus vectors for gene transfer in vivo. *Proceedings of the National Academy of Sciences of the United States of America*, **93**: 11319–20.

Markowitz, D., Goff, S. and Bank, A. (1988). A safe packaging line for gene transfer: separating viral genes on two different plasmids. *Journal of Virology*, **62**: 1120–4.

McCarty, D. M. and Samulski, R. J. (1996). Adeno-associated virus vectors for gene transfer into erythroid cells. *Current Topics in Microbiology and Immunology*, **218**: 75–91.

McKeon, C. and Samulski, R. J. (1996). NIDDK Workshop on AAV Vectors: Gene Transfer into Quiescent Cells. *Human Gene Therapy*, **7**: 1615–19.

Michael, S. I., Huang, C. H., Romer, M. U., Wagner, E., Hu, P. C. and Curiel, D. T. (1993). Binding-incompetent adenovirus facilitates molecular conjugate-mediated gene transfer by the receptor-mediated endocytosis pathway. *Journal of Biological Chemistry*, **268**: 6866–9.

Miller, A. D. and Chen, F. (1996). Retrovirus packaging cells based on 10A1 murine leukemia virus for production of vectors that use multiple receptors for cell entry. *Journal of Virology*, **70**: 5564–71.

Miller, D. G., Adam, M. A. and Miller, A. D. (1990). Gene transfer by retrovirus vectors occurs only in cells that are actively replicating at the time of infection. *Molecular and Cellular Biology*, **10**: 4239–42.

Mizukami, H., Young, N. S. and Brown, K. E. (1996). Adeno-associated virus type 2 binds to a 150-kilodalton cell membrane glycoprotein. *Virology*, **217**: 124–30.

Moss, B. (1991). Vaccinia virus: a tool for research and vaccine development. *Science*, **252**: 1662–7.

Moss, B., Carroll, M. W., Wyatt, L. S., Bennink, J. R., Hirsch, V. M., Goldstein, S., Elkins, W. R., Fuerst, T. R., Lifson, J. D., Piatak, M. and Restifo, N. P. (1996). Host range restricted, non-replicating vaccinia virus vectors as vaccine candidates. *Advances in Experimental Medical Biology*, **397**: 7–13.

Mucke, S., Polack, A., Pawlita, M., Zehnpfennig, D., Massoudi, N., Bohlen, H., Doerfler, W., Bornkamm, G., Diehl, V. and Wolf, J. (1997). Suitability of Epstein –Barr virus-based episomal vectors for expression of cytokine genes in human lymphoma cells. *Gene Therapy*, **4**: 82–92.

Mule, J. J., Custer, M., Averbook, B., Yang, J. C., Weber, J. S., Goeddel, D. V., Rosenberg, S. A. and Schall, T. J. (1996). RANTES secretion by gene-modified tumor cells results in loss of tumorigenicity in vivo: role of immune cell subpopulations. *Human Gene Therapy*, **7**: 1545–53.

Mulligan, R. C. (1993). The basic science of gene therapy. *Science*, **260**: 926–32.

Nabel, G. J., Gordon, D., Bishop, D. K., Nickoloff, B. J., Yang, Z. Y., Aruga, A., Cameron, M. J., Nabel, E. G. and Chang, A. E. (1996). Immune response in human melanoma after transfer of an allogeneic class I major histocompatibility complex gene with DNA–liposome complexes. *Proceedings of the National Academy of Sciences of the United States of America*, **93**: 15388–93.

Naldini, L., Blomer, U., Gallay, P., Ory, D., Mulligan, R., Gage, F. H., Verma, I. M. and Trono, D. (1996). In vivo gene delivery and stable transduction of nondividing cells by a lentiviral vector. *Science*, **272**: 263–7.

Naviaux, R. K., Costanzio, E., Haas, M. and Verma, I. M. (1996). The pCL vector system: rapid production of helper-free, high-titer, recombinant retroviruses. *Journal of Virology*, **70**: 5701–05.

Nguyen, D. M., Spitz, F. R., Yen, N., Cristiano, R. J. and Roth, J. A. (1996). Gene therapy for lung cancer: enhancement of tumor suppression by a combination of sequential systemic cisplatin and adenovirus-mediated p53 gene transfer. *Journal of Thoracic and Cardiovascular Surgery*, **112**: 1372–6.

Ory, D. S., Neugeboren, B. A. and Mulligan, R. C. (1996). A stable human-derived packaging cell line for production of high titer retrovirus/vesicular stomatitis virus G pseudotypes. *Proceedings of the National Academy of Sciences of the United States of America*, **93**: 11400–6.

Paoletti, E. (1996). Applications of pox virus vectors to vaccination: an update. *Proceedings of the National Academy of Sciences of the United States of America*, **93**: 11349–53.

Parks, R. J., Chen, L., Anton, M., Sankar, U., Rudnicki, M. A. and Graham, F. L. (1996). A helper-dependent adenovirus vector system: removal of helper virus by Cre-mediated excision of the viral packaging signal. *Proceedings of the National Academy of Sciences of the United States of America*, **93**: 13565–70.

Peel, A. L., Zolotukhin, S., Schrimsher, G. W., Muzyczka, N. and Reier, P. J. (1997). Efficient transduction of green fluorescent protein in spinal cord neurons using adeno-associated virus vectors containing cell type-specific promoters. *Gene Therapy*, **4**: 16–24.

Pensiero, M. N., Wysocki, C. A., Nader, K. and Kikuchi, G. E. (1996). Development of amphotropic murine retrovirus vectors resistant to inactivation by human serum. *Human Gene Therapy*, **7**: 1095–101.

Pertmer, T. M., Eisenbraun, M. D., McCabe, SD., Prayaga, S. K., Fuller, D. H. and Haynes, J. R. (1995). Gene gun-based nucleic acid immunization: elicitation of humoral and cytotoxic T lymphocyte responses following epidermal delivery of nanogram quantities of DNA. *Vaccine*, **13**: 1427–30.

Plank, C., Zatloukal, K., Cotten, M., Mechtler, K. and Wagner, E. (1992). gene transfer into hepatocytes using asialoglycoprotein receptor mediated endocytosis of DNA complexed with an artificial tetra-antennary galactose ligand. *Bioconjugate Chemistry*, **3**: 533–9.

Poeschla, E., Corbeau, P. and Wong-Staal, F. (1996). Development of HIV vectors for anti-HIV gene therapy. *Proceedings of the National Academy of Sciences of the United States of America*, **93**: 11395–9.

Qazilbash, M. H., Xiao, X., Seth, P., Cowan, K. H. and Walsh, C. E. (1997). Cancer gene therapy using a novel adeno-associated virus vector expressing human wild-type p53. *Gene Therapy*, **4**: 675–82.

Qiu, P., Ziegelhoffer, P., Sun, J. and Yang, N. S. (1996). Gene gun delivery of mRNA in situ results in efficient transgene expression and genetic immunization. *Gene Therapy*, **3**: 262–8.

Rakhmilevich, A. L., Turner, J., Ford, M. J., McCabe, D., Sun, W. H., Sondel, P. M., Grota, K. and Yang, N. S. (1996). Gene gun-mediated skin transfection with interleukin 12 gene results in regression of established primary and metastatic murine tumors. *National Academy of Sciences of the United States of America*, **93**: 6291–6.

Ram, Z., Walbridge, S., Heiss, J. D., Culver, K. W., Blaese, R. M. and Oldfield, E. H. (1994a). In vivo transfer of the human interleukin-2 gene: negative tumoricidal results in experimental brain tumors. *Journal of Neurosurgery*, **80**: 535–40.

Ram, Z., Walbridge, S., Shawker, T., Culver, K. W., Blaese, R. M. and Oldfield, E. H. (1994b). The effect of thymidine kinase transduction and ganciclovir therapy on tumor vasculature and growth of 9L gliomas in rats. *Journal of Neurosurgery*, **81**: 256–60.

Ratliff, T. L., Kawakita, M., Tartaglia, J. and Paoletti, E. (1996). Canary-pox (ALVAC) virus-mediated cytokine gene therapy induces tumor specific and non-specific immunity against mouse prostate tumor. *Acta Urologica Belgica*, **64**: 85.

Richards, C. A., Austin, E. A. and Huber, B. E. (1995). Transcriptional regulatory sequences of carcinoembryonic antigen: identification and use with cytosine deaminase for tumor-specific gene therapy. *Human Gene Therapy*, **6**: 881–93.

Roth, J., Dittmer, D., Rea, D., Tartaglia, J., Paoletti, E. and Levine, A. J. (1996). p53 as a target for cancer vaccines: recombinant canarypox virus vectors expressing p53 protect mice against lethal tumor cell challenge. *Proceedings of the National Academy of Sciences of the United States of America*, **93**: 4781–6.

Samulski, R. J., Zhu, X., Xiao, X., Brook, J. D., Housman, D. E., Epstein, N. and Hunter, L. A. (1991). Targeted integration of adeno-associated virus (AAV) into human chromosome 19. *EMBO Journal*, **10**: 3941–50.

Sanda, M. G., Ayyagari, S. R., Jaffee, E. M., Epstein, J. I., Clift, S. L., Cohen, L. K., Dranoff, G., Pardoll, D. M., Mulligan, R. C. and Simons, J. W. (1994). Demonstration of a rational strategy for human prostate cancer gene therapy. *Journal of Urology*, **151**: 622–8.

Schwarzenberger, P., Spence, S. E., Gooya, J. M., Michiel, D., Curiel, D. T., Ruscetti, F. W. and Keller, J. R. (1996). Targeted gene transfer to human hematopoietic progenitor cell lines through the c-kit receptor. *Blood*, **87**: 472–8.

Seth, P. (1994a). Adenovirus-dependent release of choline from plasma membrane vesicles at an acidic pH is mediated by the penton base protein. *Journal of Virology*, **68**: 1204–06.

Seth, P. (1994b). Mechanism of adenovirus-mediated endosome lysis: role of the intact adenovirus capsid structure. *Biochemical and Biophysical Research Communications*, **205**: 1318–24.

Seth, P. (1994c). A simple and efficient method of protein delivery into cells using adenovirus. *Biochemical and Biophysical Research Communications*, **203**: 582–7.

Seth, P., Fitzgerald, D., Ginsberg, H., Willingham, M. and Pastan, I. (1986). Pathway of adenovirus entry into cells. In R. Crowell and K. Lonberg-Holm (eds.), *Virus attachment and entry into cells*, pp. 191–5. American Society for Microbiology, Washington, D.C.

Seth, P., Rosenfeld, M., Higginbotham, J. and Crystal, R. G. (1994). Mechanism of enhancement of DNA expression consequent to cointernalization of a replication-deficient adenovirus and unmodified plasmid DNA. *Journal of Virology*, **68**: 933–40.

Seth, P., Brinkmann, U., Schwartz, G. N., Katayose, D., Gress, R., Pastan, I. and Cowan, K. (1996). Adenovirus-mediated gene transfer to human breast tumor cells: an approach for cancer gene therapy and bone marrow purging. *Cancer Research*, **56**: 1346–51.

Seth, P., Katayose, D., Craig, C., Li, Z., Ohri, E., Kim, M., Wersto, R., Mudasar, B., Rakkar, A., Kodali, P. and Cowan, K. (1997). A recombinant adenovirus expressing wild type p53 induces apoptosis in drug resistant breast cancer cells: a gene therapy approach for drug resistant cancers. *Cancer Gene Therapy*, **4**: 383–90.

Shenk, T. (1996). Adenoviridae: The viruses and their replication. In B. N. Fields, D. M. Knippe and P. Howley (eds.) *Fields Virology*, pp. 2111–48. Lippincot-Raven, Philadelphia.

Simons, J. W., Jaffee, E. M., Weber, C. E., Levitsky, H. I., Nelson, W. G., Carducci, M. A., Lazenby, A. J., Cohen, L. K., Finn, C. C., Clift, S. M. and Hauda, K. M. (1997). Bioactivity of autologous irradiated renal cell carcinoma vaccines generated by ex vivo granulocyte–macrophage colony-stimulating factor gene transfer. *Cancer Research*, **57**: 1537–46.

Somia, N. V., Zoppe, M. and Verma, I. M. (1995). Generation of targeted retroviral vectors by using single-chain variable fragment: an approach to in vivo gene delivery. *Proceedings of the National Academy of Sciences of the United States of America*, **92**: 7570–4.

Spitz, F. R., Nguyen, D., Skibber, J. M., Cusack, J., Roth, J. A. and Cristiano, R. J. (1996). In vivo adenovirus-mediated p53 tumor suppressor gene therapy for colorectal cancer. *Anticancer Research*, **16**: 3415–22.

Stratford-Perricaudet, L. D., Makeh, I., Perricaudet, M. and Briand, P. (1992). Widespread long-term gene transfer to mouse skeletal muscles and heart. *Journal of Clinical Investigation*, **90**: 626–30.

Sun, W. H., Burkholder, J. K., Sun, J., Culp, J., Turner, J., Lu, X. G., Pugh, T. D., Ershler, W. B. and Yang, N. S. (1995). In vivo cytokine gene transfer by gene gun reduces tumor growth in mice. *Proceedings of the National Academy of Sciences of the United States of America*, **92**: 2889–93.

Takahara, Y., Hamada, K. and Housman, D. E. (1992). A new retrovirus packaging cell for gene transfer constructed from amplified long terminal repeat-free chimeric proviral genes. *Journal of Virology*, **66**: 3725–32.

Tanaka, T., Kanai, F., Okabe, S., Yoshida, Y., Wakimoto, H., Hamada, H., Shiratori, Y., Lan, K., Ishitobi, M. and Omata, M. (1996). Adenovirus-mediated prodrug gene therapy for carcinoembryonic antigen-producing human gastric carcinoma cells in vitro. *Cancer Research*, **56**: 1341–5.

Torres, C. A., Wasaki, A., Barber, B. H. and Robinson, H. L. (1997). Differential dependence on target site tissue for gene gun and intramuscular DNA immunizations. *Journal of Immunology*, **158**: 4529–32.

Trempe, J. P. (1996). Packaging systems for adeno-associated virus vectors. *Current Topics in Microbiology and Immunology*, **218**: 35–50.

Trinh, Q. T., Austin, E. A., Murray, D. M., Knick, V. C. and Huber, B. E. (1995). Enzyme/prodrug gene therapy: comparison of cytosine deaminase/5-fluorocytosine versus thymidine kinase/ganciclovir enzyme/prodrug systems in a human colorectal carcinoma cell line. *Cancer Research*, **55**: 4808–12.

Verma, I. M. (1994). Gene therapy: hopes, hypes, and hurdles. *Molecular Medicine*, **1**: 2–3.

Vile, R. G. (1996). Gene therapy for cancer, the course ahead. *Cancer Metastasis Reviews*, **15**: 403–10.

Vile, R., Miller, N., Chernajovsky, Y. and Hart, I. (1994). A comparison of the properties of different retroviral vectors containing the murine tyrosinase promoter to achieve transcriptionally targeted expression of the HSVtk or IL-2 genes. *Gene Therapy*, **1**: 307–16.

Vile, R. G., Diaz, R. M., Miller, N., Mitchell, S., Tuszyanski, A. and Russell, S. J. (1995). Tissue-specific gene expression from Mo-MLV retroviral vectors with hybrid LTRs containing the murine tyrosinase enhancer/promoter. *Virology*, **214**: 307–13.

Vile, R. G., Tuszynski, A. and Castleden, S. (1996). Retroviral vectors. From laboratory tools to molecular medicine. *Molecular Biotechnology*, **5**: 139–58.

Wang, H., Kavanaugh, M. P., North, R. A. and Kabat, D. (1991). Cell-surface receptor for ecotropic murine retroviruses is a basic amino-acid transporter. *Nature*, **352**: 729–31.

Wang, X. S., Ponnazhagan, S. and Srivastava, A. (1996). Rescue and replication of adeno-associated virus type 2 as well as vector DNA sequences from recombinant plasmids containing deletions in the viral inverted terminal repeats: selective encapsidation of viral genomes in progeny virions. *Journal of Virology*, **70**: 1668–77.

Wolff, J. A., Malone, R. W., Williams, P., Chong, W., Acsadi, G., Jani, A. and Felgner, P. L. (1990). Direct gene transfer into mouse muscle in vivo. *Science*, **247**: 1465–8.

Xu, X., Dai, Y., Heidenreich, O. and Nerenberg, M. I. (1996). Adenovirus-mediated interferon-gamma transfer inhibits growth of transplanted HTLV-1 Tax tumors in mice. *Human Gene Therapy*, **7**: 741–7.

Yagi, K., Hayashi, Y., Ishida, N., Ohbayashi, M., Ohishi, N., Mizuno, M. and Yoshida, J. (1994). Interferon-beta endogenously produced by intratumoral injection of cationic liposome-encapsulated gene: cytocidal effect on glioma transplanted into nude mouse brain. *Biochemistry Molecular Biology International*, **32**: 167–71.

Yajima, H., Kosukegawa, A., Hoque, M. M. et al. (1996). Construction and characterization of a recombinant adenovirus vector carrying the human preproinsulin gene under the control of the metallothionein gene promoter. *Biochemical and Biophysical Research Communications*, **229**: 778–87.

Yang, N. S. and Sun, W. H. (1995). Gene gun and other non-viral approaches for cancer gene therapy. *Nature Medicine*, **1**: 481–3.

Yang, Y., Greenough, K. and Wilson, J. M. (1996). Transient immune blockade prevents formation of neutralizing antibody to recombinant adenovirus and allows repeated gene transfer to mouse liver. *Gene Therapy*, **3**: 412–20.

Yee, J. K., Friedman, T. and Burns, J. C. (1994). Generation of high-titer pseudotyped retroviral vectors with very broad host range. *Methods in Cell Biology*, **43**: 99–112.

Yoshimura, K., Rosenfeld, M. A., Seth, P. and Crystal, R. G. (1993). Adenovirus-mediated augmentation of cell transfection with unmodified plasmid vectors. *Journal of Biological Chemistry*, **268**: 2300–3.

Zhang, W. W. (1996). Growth inhibitory effect of anti-K-ras adenovirus on lung cancer cells. *Cancer Gene Therapy*, **3**: 296–301.

Zhang, Y., Mukhopadhyay, T., Donehower, L. A., Georges, R. N. and Roth, J. A. (1993). Retroviral vector-mediated transduction of K-ras antisense RNA into human lung cancer cells inhibits expression of the malignant phenotype. *Human Gene Therapy*, **4**: 451–60.

4

Genetically engineering drug sensitivity and drug resistance for the treatment of cancer

BRIAN E. HUBER

Chemotherapy and therapeutic selectivity

In selected cases, chemotherapy targeted against many infectious agents has proven to be both extremely safe and efficacious. In these cases, therapeutic selectivity is achieved by exploiting *qualitative* differences in the structure, function, or intermediary metabolism between the target organism and the human cells.

Structural

Certain very safe and effective antibiotics therapeutically exploit the fact that bacteria require intact cell walls to maintain their integrity. Certain antibiotics can disrupt the formation or the integrity of the cell wall, causing the invading bacterium to become fragile and ultimately lyse. For example, peptidoglycan is a highly crosslinked, heteropolymeric component of the cell wall which is the molecular basis for its rigid structure. It is composed of linear chains of alternating units of N-acetylglucosamine and N-acetylmuramic acid which are linked by peptide crosslinks. The final phase of peptidoglycan synthesis is the crosslinking of the glycopeptide polymers by a transpeptidase reaction which occurs on the outside of the bacterial cell membrane. It appears that this transpeptidase step is inhibited by the beta-lactam antibiotics, such as the penicillins (i.e., penicillin G, V, ampicillin, oxacillin, etc.) and cephalosporins (i.e., cephapirin, cephalexin, cefaclor, cefotaxime, etc.). The beta-lactam antibiotics also bind to other bacteria-specific proteins (called penicillin-binding proteins, or PBP), which may significantly contribute to their antibacterial effects. Inhibition of the cell wall transpeptidase reaction and PBP binding causes the bacteria to lyse due to the autolytic activity of autolysins and murein hydrolases located in the cell wall.

Functional

Bacteria have specific ribosomal components which are qualitatively distinct from eukaryotic ribosomes. The aminoglycoside antibiotics (i.e., gentamycin, streptomycin, neomycin, etc.) appear to exert their selective bacterial toxicity by binding to the 30S component of the bacterial ribosome. Binding is then followed by disruption of initiation of protein synthesis and perhaps misreading of the RNA template, causing misincorporation of amino acids.

Intermediary metabolism

Certain enzymes have exquisite substrate specificities that can be therapeutically exploited. Bacterial and viral enzymes can have substrate specificities that qualitatively and/or quantitatively differ from their mammalian counterparts. For example, acyclovir and gancyclovir have been shown to be very effective and selective agents for herpes simplex-1 virus (HSV-1). This was demonstrated to be the result of a virus-specific thymidine kinase gene. Acyclovir and gancyclovir are approximately 200-fold better substrates for the herpes simplex virus thymidine kinase (HSV TK) compared to the mammalian thymidine kinase (Elion et al., 1978; Fyfe, et al., 1978; Elion, 1982). The first phosphorylation step takes place at a negligble rate in uninfected mammalian cells. However, once monophosphorylated in virally infected cells, other mammalian kinases can further anabolize acyclovir and gancyclovir to the diphosphate and triphosphate level (Figure 4.1). Hence, the selective anabolism of acyclovir and gancyclovir to the active triphosophate is dependent upon the first monophosphorylation step performed by the herpes-specific TK. Additional selectively is achieved at the DNA polymerase level as well, since acyclovir–triphosphate also interferes with the DNA polymerase. Once acyclovir or gancyclovir is anabolized to the triphosphate level, it interferes with DNA synthesis, which ultimately leads to death of the virally infected cell.

Another example of selectivity being dependent upon selective metabolism is the very safe and effective antifungal agent 5-fluorocytosine (5-FC). This compound is not metabolized to any significant degree by mammalian cells, and therefore remains inert and nontoxic. However, certain fungi (e.g., *Cryptococcus*, *Candida*, *Torulopsis*, etc.) contain a specific anabolic enzyme, cytosine deaminase, which is not found in mammalian cells. This enzyme can very selectively convert 5-FC to the toxic agent, 5 fluorouracil (5-FU), in the fungal cells (Figure 4.2). Once 5-FU is generated, it will inhibit cell division by inhibition of thymidylate synthetase and possibly by incorporation into RNA.

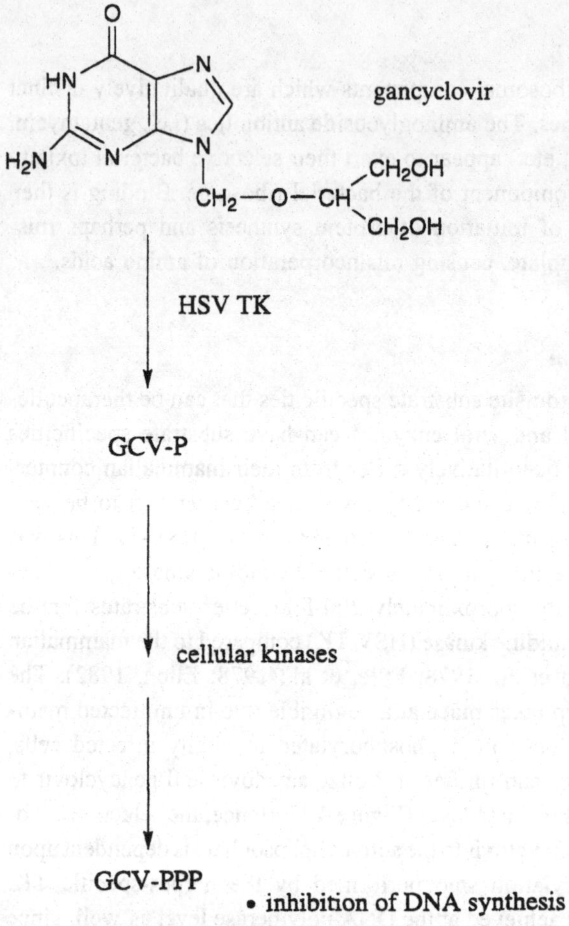

Fig. 4.1. Gancyclovir anabolism.

Cancer chemotherapy

Unlike chemotherapy targeted at infectious organisms, chemotherapy targeted at neoplastic disease has generally relied upon more subtle quantitative biochemical differences between normal and neoplastic cells to achieve therapeutic selectivity. To date, many of the marginally effective antineoplastic compounds have been mechanistically dependent upon dividing versus nondividing cells as the basis for selectively. Lack of exploitable qualitative biochemical differences in neoplastic cells has resulted in marginally effective,

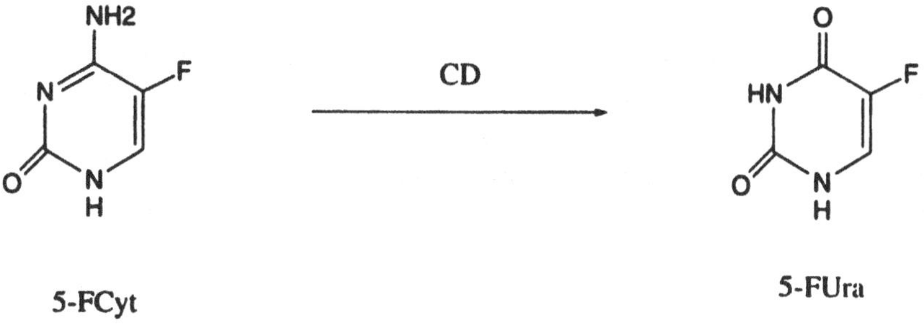

Fig. 4.2. 5-FC metabolism.

systemically toxic therapies. Efficacy has been continually improved with traditional cytotoxic agents by:

- utilizing multiple drug combinations;
- identification of better pharmacokinetic dosing regimens with appropriate recovery times for normal cells;
- use of biological-response modifiers to reduce systemic toxicity, allowing for dose intensification;
- addition of immunomodulatory agents.

There are specific examples where cellular transformation may be initiated and maintained by transforming proteins which may have qualitative biochemical differences compared to their normal counterparts. An example of this is the mutated *ras* oncogene. However, these specific, qualitatively altered proteins have yet to be meaningfully exploited therapeutically. Due to the inherent lack of selectivity, traditional cancer chemotherapy has proved to have significant side-effects and is only marginally effective for the vast majority of major solid tumors. It is obvious that novel approaches for cancer therapy are still needed.

Gene therapy

Gene therapy has been defined in various ways (for example see Anderson, 1984; Miller, 1990). A broad, encompassing definition of human gene therapy is the in-vivo or ex-vivo transfer of defined genetic material to specific target cells of a patient, thereby altering the genotype and, in most situations, altering the phenotype of those target cells for the ultimate purpose of preventing or altering a particular disease state. As this definition states, the underlying premise is that these *therapeutic* genetic procedures are designed ultimately to prevent, treat, or alter an overt or covert pathological condition. In most situations, the ultimate therapeutic goal of gene therapy procedures will be to alter the phenotype of a specific target cell population. However, there may be particular medical situations, such as in latent disease states, where the therapeutic goal will only be to alter the genotype of a particular target cell population before the occurrence of any overt pathological condition.

Chapter 1 in this book summarizes the evolution and applications of gene therapy approaches for the treatment of cancer. The remainder of this chapter describes the progress and prospects of genetically engineering drug sensitivity or drug resistance for more effective ways to treat neoplastic disease.

Enzyme/prodrug gene therapy for the treatment of solid tumors

Many different laboratories and clinical centers have been developing novel gene therapy approaches for cancer therapy that involve selectively creating qualitative biochemical differences between normal and neoplastic cells. The basic principle of these approaches is the transduction of a chimeric gene composed of a tumor-associated transcriptional regulatory sequence (TRS) linked to the protein-coding domain encoding a nonhuman enzyme. Since expression of the nonhuman enzyme is controlled by the tumor-associated TRS, the nonhuman enzyme will be selectively expressed in the tumor mass, thus generating a qualitative biochemical difference between the tumor cells and the adjacent normal cells. The nonhuman enzyme can selectively 'activate' or convert a nontoxic prodrug into an 'active' toxic metabolite, thus killing the cancer cell. The selectivity of these approaches relies on the selective delivery, expression or function of the nonhuman enzyme in the cancer cell and/or the selective delivery or activation of the nontoxic prodrug to the active metabolite in the cancer cell. The term that has been used to describe this enzyme/prodrug approach is virus-directed enzyme/prodrug therapy (VDEPT).

Backdrop and historical development of enzmye/produg gene therapy

The concept and clinical development of enzyme/prodrug gene therapy have comprised a completely novel application of gene therapy for the treatment of cancer. Before the advent of gene therapy, this approach could not have been attempted due to the fundamental requirement of in-vivo gene transfer. However, like all novel discoveries, the concept of enzyme/prodrug gene therapy for the treatment of cancer can be linked to seemingly unrelated observations in other fields, namely mechanistic studies involving the antiviral agents, acyclovir and gancyclovir.

To verify the mechanism of acyclovir and confirm that the *HSV TK* gene is the sole, specific element responsible for the first selective anabolic activation step of acyclovir activation, HSV DNA-encoding *HSV TK* was transfected into cells (Furman et al., 1980; Davidson et al., 1981; Kucera, Furman and Elion, 1983; St Clair, Lambe and Furman, 1987). Data generated from these transfected cells confirmed that the *HSV TK* gene is the only required viral gene for activation of acyclovir. More importantly, these transfected cells confirmed that the viral *TK* gene is absolutely required for the efficient metabolic activation of acyclovir to a cytotoxic anabolite.

The *HSV TK* gene has also been used as a reporter gene in the creation of transgenic animals. The mouse mammary tumor virus long terminal repeat was linked to the *HSV TK* gene and transgenic animals were created using this construct (Ross and Solter, 1985). However, in this case, the unique and specific biochemical properties of HSV TK were not utilized or taken advantage of. In this particular case, *HSV TK* was used only as a marker gene to be detected by Southern and northern blot analysis and by HSV TK protein levels. The real value of the *HSV TK* gene lies in its unique and selective biochemical substrate requirements. In developmental biology studies, a key issue is the ability to understand the interdependence and linkage between different cell types. To help address some of these key cell lineage issues, the *HSV TK* gene has been used to conditionally ablate certain cell lineages in transgenic animals by using relevant promoter and enhancer sequences to selectively express the *HSV TK* gene. This was first accomplished by conditionally ablating B-cell and T-cell lineages by fusing the *HSV TK*-coding sequence to the mouse immunoglobulin μ heavy-chain enhancer and the mouse $\varkappa$ light chain promoter (Borelli et al., 1988; Heyman, et al., 1989). Another example of this approach is the study of growth hormone and prolactin-producing cells of the anterior pituitary gland. Transgenic animals were created using the *HSV TK* gene under the transcriptional control of either the rat growth hormone or rat prolactin promoter and enhancer sequences (Borrelli et al., 1989). Although these studies showed the value of using the *HSV TK* gene to ablate specific cell populations in cell lineage and developmental biology studies, they utilized transgenic animal technology which has no therapeutic applicability.

Mosaicism and the prophylactic control of cancer

The first *theoretical* application for the therapeutic use of genetically expressing a nonhuman enzyme for the treatment of cancer was proposed by Moolten. Moolten proposed to control cancer prophylactically or prospectively by creating genetically mosaic individuals (Moolten, 1976; for review see Moolten, 1990). The Moolten hypothesis was as follows. Genes which can specifically alter the cellular sensitivity to various agents are randomly introduced into all the tissues and cells of healthy patients in a prophylactic manner. In a particular tissue, some cells will possess gene A, others gene B and others gene X. Hence, mosaic individuals are created prospectively to permit the control of future cancer. If a cancer arises at a future date, it is characterized as to which sensitivity gene it expresses. Treatment is then based on this mosaic expression pattern. Many different sensitivity genes could be utilized, including genes which can activate prodrugs, inhibitors of drug-resistance genes, transcription factors, etc.

Of course, technical issues prevent even the laboratory testing of the mosaic hypothesis. Assuming that all cancers are clonal in nature, this mosaic hypothesis assumes that multiple gene transfers can be conducted in all somatic cells of the body so that each cell has a different complement of multiply-transduced sensitivity genes. These genes would then need to be expressed or transcriptionally activated decades after the original gene transfers. Cell turnover would necessitate that all pluripotent stem cells receive a different complement of drug-sensitivity genes. If drug-resistance genes were also used, as originally suggested, then all normal cells surrounding the tumor and all normal cells subject to toxicity (but not the cancer cells) must express this resistance gene. These are but a few of the technical issues which will prevent the evaluation and development of the mosaic hypothesis.

VDEPT and GDEPT

More realistic efforts have been proposed that exploit the use of enzyme/prodrug therapy. Many of these proposals have been preclinically tested as well as being clinically evaluated. The exploitation of enzyme/prodrug therapy for the treatment of solid tumors has been practically developed by VDEPT (Moolten and Wells, 1990; Huber, Richards and Krenitsky, 1991; Culver et al., 1992; Mullen, Kilstrup and Blaese, 1992; Austin and Huber, 1993; Huber et al., 1993, 1994). This approach was originally developed for use with viral gene-delivery vectors. Since other, nonviral, gene-delivery vectors can be used as well, this approach has more recently been called GDEPT (gene-

● Creation of an artificial gene for gene therapy

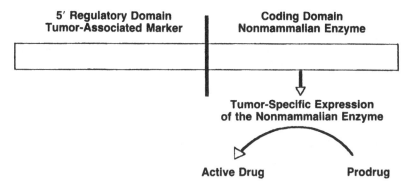

Fig. 4.3. Virus-directed enzyme/prodrug therapy strategy.

directed enzyme/prodrug therapy). The VDEPT approach exploits the transcriptional differences between normal and neoplastic cells to selectively kill the cancer cells. An artificial, chimeric gene is created that is composed of a tissue-specific TRS linked to the protein-coding domain of a nonhuman enzyme. The nonhuman enzyme metabolically activates a nontoxic prodrug to a cytotoxic anabolite. If the TRS is from a tumor-associated gene, such as carcinoembryonic antigen (CEA), then the artificial gene will produce tumor-associated expression of the nonhuman enzyme and, consequently, tumor-associated production of the cytotoxic anabolite (Figure 4.3).

To date, HSV TK/gancyclovir and CD/5-FC have been the most utilized enzyme/prodrug combinations to be utilized in the VDEPT approach. However, many other enzyme systems have been proposed and are in various stages of preclinical evaluation. Some of these enzyme/prodrug combinations are identified in Table 4.1

To achieve tumor-selective expression of the activating enzyme, tumor-selective TRS are ultilized. These TRS are isolated from promoter and enhancer sequences of tumor-associated marker genes. In addition, TRS can be utilized in VDEPT which are actually tissue specific but are 'operationally' tumor selective. An example of a tumor type which can utilize a selective tissue-specific TRS is ovarian cancer. The primary ovarian tumor is eliminated by surgical resection. Metastatic ovarian cancer in the peritoneal cavity can be targeted with a VDEPT approach. In this particular case, TRS which are ovary specific will suffice to achieve selectivity, since the tissue of origin has been surgically removed. In other cases, tissue-specific TRS can be utilized

Table 4.1. *Enzyme/prodrug combinations that are in various stages of preclinical evaluation for VDEPT*

Enzyme	Prodrug
HSV TK	Gancyclovir
CD	5-FC
Nitroreductase	5-Aziridine 2, 4-dinitrobenzamidine
β-Lactamase (MDA)*	Phenylenediamine mustard cephalosporin
Carboxypeptidase G2 (MDA)*	Benzoic acid mustard glutamic acid
Carboxypeptidase A (MDA)*	Methotrexate-linked molecules
β-Glucosidase (MDA)*	Amygdalin

*MDA = multidrug activation system. Many different enzymes will cleave a standard chemical linkage. Due to this property, many different prodrugs can be formulated using this standard linkage. Only one is shown for each enzyme.

Table 4.2. *Transcription regulatory sequences that can be utilized in the VDEPT approach*

Transcriptional regulatory sequence	Tumor
Carcinoembryonic antigen (CEA)	Colorectal, lung, breast, gastric
Alpha-fetoprotein (AFP)	Heptaocellular carcinoma
Prostate-specific antigen (PSA)	Prostate
Glial fibrillary acid protein	Glioma
c-erb B2	Breast
Neuroendocrine markers	Lung and gastric
Tyrosinase	Melanoma

if normal tissues that are capable of expressing the marker gene will not be exposed to the vector or TRS are derived from tissues that can tolerate toxicity (Table 4.2). In addition to tumor-associated TRS, TRS isolated from genes transcriptionally induced by radiation have also been used in the VDEPT approach (Weichselbaum et al., 1992; Khil et al., 1996).

There are many levels of therapeutic selectivity in the VDEPT approach (Table 4.3). A first level of tumor selectivity can be achieved by local or regional delivery of the gene-transfer vector. The vector may be directly administered to the tumor mass by direct intralesional injection (see below). Certain tumors may be confined to discrete 'compartments,' such as the peritoneal cavity, bladder, pleural space, etc. The gene-transfer vector can be specifically administered to this 'isolated' site so that the vector has direct access to the tumor. Differences in regional blood supply can also be exploited.

Table 4.3. *Selectivity in VDEPT*

1. Physical administration of the gene-transfer vector:
   direct intralesional injection
   'isolated' compartmentalization
   exploitation of differences in blood flow
2. Properties of the gene-transfer vector
3. Selective expression of the nonhuman, drug-activating enzyme
4. Selective metabolic activation of the prodrug
5. Selectivity generated by the specific intermediary metabolism

Tumors in certain organs have distinct differences in blood supply compared to the normal cells of that organ. An excellent example of this is the distinct differences in blood supply of the normal cells in the liver compared to primary or metastatic tumors in the liver. Normal hepatic parenchyma cells receive their blood supply predominantly from the portal vein. Primary and metastatic tumors in the liver (along with the biliary system) receive their blood supply predominantly from the hepatic artery. Hence, by infusing the vector into the hepatic artery, the tumor is perfused to a much greater extent than the normal liver parenchyma cells.

Another level of selectivity in VDEPT can be realized by taking advantage of the specific properties of the gene-transfer vectors. Murine retroviral gene-transfer vectors require the target cells to be in cycle and synthesizing DNA for the vector to integrate and express (Miller, Adam and Miller, 1990). Certain organs, such as the brain, are characterized by predominantly non-dividing cell populations. These two properties can be effectively exploited in VDEPT targeting primary or metastatic brain tumors (Culver et al., 1992). Other vectors, such as adenoviral vectors or HIV-based vectors, may have tissue tropisms (liver and specific T cell populations, respectively) that may eventually be exploited to achieve a level of selectivity.

A major level of selectivity in VDEPT is achieved by the selective expression of the nonhuman prodrug-activating enzyme in tumor cells. The use of transcriptional regulatory sequences of tumor-associated marker genes to express the nonhuman enzyme will restrict expression of the nonhuman enzyme to tumor cells which express the tumor-associated marker. This has been successfully exploited in preclinical studies using the tumor-associated markers for colorectal cancer (CEA) and hepatocellular carcinoma (alpha-fetoprotein). Many other tumors have very restricted expression of specific tumor markers that can be exploited in VEDPT. Although some of these markers may not make good primary diagnostic markers for cancer since they

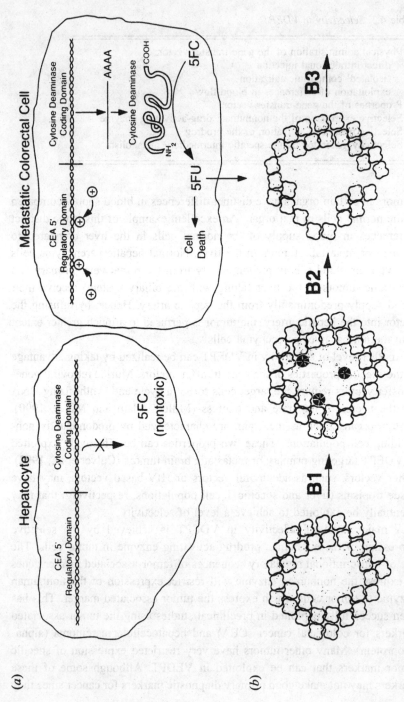

Fig. 4.4. Suicide gene therapy for colon cancer.

are expressed at later stages in the development of malignant disease, they will provide excellent transcriptional regulatory sequences for VDEPT.

Finally, selectivity for the tumor mass can be achieved via the inherent biochemical and intermediary metabolism of the tumor and surrounding tissues. An excellent example of this is the use of the cytosine deaminase (*CD*) gene for the VDEPT treatment approach for metastatic colorectal tumors contained within the liver compartment. As cited above, cytosine deaminase catalyzes the conversion of cytosine and 5-FC to uracil and 5-FU, respectively (Figure 4.2). *CD* has been effectively utilized in a VDEPT approach for metastatic colorectal cancer (Figure 4.4). It can be selectively expressed in metastatic colorectal tumor cells in the liver compartment by using the CEA transcriptional regulatory sequence. Once expressed, *CD* can convert the nontoxic prodrug, 5-FC, to the toxic anabolite, 5-FU. The first step in the catabolism of 5-FU is catalyzed by the enzyme uracil reductase. Colorectal tumor cells have very little uracil reductase activity, so 5-FU has a relatively long half-life in these cells. Hepatocytes, on the other hand, have very high levels of uracil reductase. Hence, any 5-FU that diffuses out of the metastatic colorectal tumor cells and into the normal liver compartment will be immediately catabolized by uracil reductase. This aspect of specific biochemical properties and intermediary metabolism adds to the level of selectivity in the VDEPT approach.

A VDEPT approach that incorporates all levels of selectivity is that proposed by Huber et al. (Huber et al., 1993, 1994; Austin and Huber, 1993), for the treatment of metastatic colorectal cancer in the liver compartment. In this particular system, the retroviral vector is administered into the liver via the hepatic artery to perfuse the tumor to a greater extent than normal hepatic parenchyma cells. The retroviral vector has a much greater propensity to infect dividing tumor cells rather than the nondividing hepatocytes. The chimeric gene delivered by the retroviral vector is composed of the CEA TRS driving expression of the *CD*-coding domain. This will limit expression to CEA-positive cells of the tumor. Tumor-selective expression of *CD* will permit the selective conversion of 5-FC to 5-FU at the tumor site. 5-FU can diffuse throughout the tumor mass by nonfacilitated diffusion. Any 5-FU that diffuses into the normal liver compartment will be immediately catabolized by uracil reductase located in the hepatocyte.

All levels of selectivity are not required to achieve a meaningful therapeutic benefit. Some enzyme/prodrug approaches do not rely on a tissue-specific or tumor-specific promoter to express the nonhuman drug-activating enzyme. Selectivity may, for example, be achieved solely by the properties of the gene-transfer vector. For example, Culver and Blaese developed a system for the treatment of brain tumors using retroviral vectors to deliver the *HSV TK* gene to the brain tumor (Culver et al., 1992). The underlying premise behind this approach is that tumors in the brain will be composed of actively dividing cells which are subject to retroviral infection, whereas normal brain tissue is composed of essentially nondividing cells which are resistant to retroviral gene transduction. Hence, selectivity is achieved solely on the basis of the properties of the gene-delivery vector and the milieu in which the tumor is located. To enhance gene transduction efficiency, the retroviral-producing cells were injected intralesionally, rather than the retrovirus itself. These retroviral-packaging or retroviral-producing cells served as a 'viral factory' by continually producing retroviral particles in and around the tumor for approximately 24 to 72 hours. This will theoretically aid in transduction efficiency since:

- more total virus may be able to be delivered to the tumor mass;
- virus will theoretically be present at the tumor site for a greater period of time, so when an individual tumor cell enters S phase, the probability is higher that a viral particle will be present to transduce that cell.

Based on preclinical efficacy and safety data in rats (Culver et al., 1992), Recombinant DNA Advisory Committee (RAC) approved a clinical protocol submitted by these investigators to evaluate the stereotactic implantation into brain tumors of retroviral-packaging cells which produced a retrovirus containing a gene for the nonspecific expression of *HSV TK* (Oldfield et al., 1993).

A consistently encountered issue with all present gene-transduction vectors is the relatively low transduction efficiency obtained in in-vivo gene-delivery protocols. In addition, there is heterogeneity within a solid tumor mass with respect to how many cells are actively in the cell cycle as well as regarding expression of the tumor-associated marker gene. Due to these issues, antitumor efficacy in enzyme/prodrug approaches relies on bystander tumor cell-killing effects. Bystander killing effects have been measured in many enzyme/prodrug combinations and in many different cell lines and tumors. They are the result of different mechanisms, and which mechanism predominates is dependent upon the enzyme/prodrug combination and the tumor type. Bystander killing can be the result of diffusion of the toxic anabolite of the prodrug, transport of the toxic anabolite via gap junctions between cells, disruption of tumor vasculature, immunological stimulation resulting from better exposure of tumor antigens, and, potentially, release of apoptotic vesicles.

Other applications of drugs-sensitivity genes

Genetically engineering drug sensitivity via the introduction of drug-sensitivity genes has applications outside the cancer therapeutics area. One of the serious concerns regarding both ex-vivo and in-vivo gene transfer is the theoretical ability to transform cells that have been genetically altered. The concern is greatest for those gene-transfer vectors which can integrate and disrupt the integrity of the cell's genome. Retroviral transduction vectors are an example of this type of vector system. Transformation may theoretically occur by either transcriptional activation of an oncogene or genomic disruption of a tumor suppressor gene (Figure 4.5). This has been documented in one experiment where the retroviral preparation was contaminated by replication competent helper virus (Donahue et al., 1993). Another concern regarding gene therapy is the inappropriate expression level of the transduced gene. For example, could inappropriate overexpression of certain clotting factors used to correct specific hemophilia cause detrimental clots? Could expression of genes to enhance the immune system generate autoimmune disorders?

The questions of neoplastic transformation and other unwanted effects of gene transfer have been extensively debated in the RAC and US Food and Drug Administration (FDA). Inclusion of a drug-sensitivity gene in the gene-transfer vector may be one safety mechanism to address these concerns (e.g., Plautz, Nabel and Nabel, 1991).

Genetically engineering drug resistance

Some tumor types, such as leukemias, lymphomas and germ cell tumors, can be treated relatively successfully with antineoplastic drugs. However, for the major solid tumors, such as lung, breast, colon, and prostate, traditional chemotherapy is significantly less successful. The two main reasons for lack of clinical success are:

- inherent or acquired resistance to chemotherapeutic drugs by the tumor;
- systemic toxicity generated from the nontumor-selective properties of conventional antineoplastic drugs.

Increase in tumor drug exposure (exposure = concentration × time) can overcome both reasons for the lack of clinical success. In fact, it has been documented that small increases in tumor drug exposure can result in substantial gains in clinical efficacy. However, due to the lack of tumor selectivity by conventional antineoplastic agents, increases in dose exposure also result in unacceptable systemic, dose-limiting toxicity. A logical mechanism by

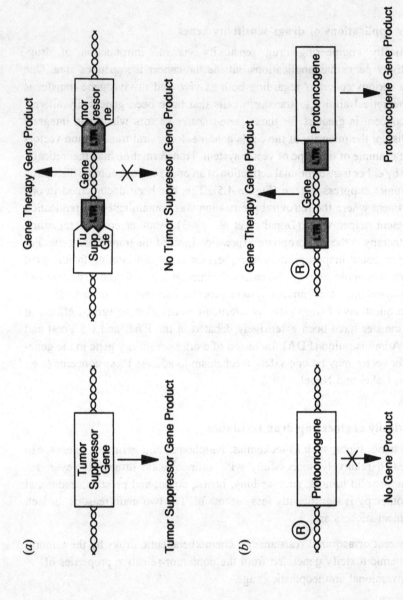

Fig. 4.5. Mechanisms of transformation by retroviruses.

which to increase tumor drug exposure is to decrease host toxicity to allow greater dosing intensity. Gene therapy approaches have allowed both preclinical (Bertolini et al., 1994; Ward et al., 1994; Flasshove et al., 1995) and initial clinical evaluation (Deisseroth, Kavanagh and Chaplin, 1994; Hesdorffer, Antman and Bank, 1994; O'Shaughnessy, Cowan and Neinhuis, 1994) of transducing drug-resistance genes into bone marrow to allow for greater dosing intensity and tumor drug exposure.

There have been a number of different drug-resistance genes identified over the last several years, some of which make good candidates for genetically engineering drug resistance. First and foremost is the multiple drug-resistance gene-1 (*MDR-1*). The *MDR-1* gene encodes a cell surface 170 kDa P-glycoprotein (gp 170). gp 170 is a cell surface efflux pump, which pumps out of cells a diverse group of lipophilic compounds such as the extensively utilized chemotherapeutic agents actinomycin D, taxol, navelbine and other vinca alkaloids, anthracyclines, and epipodophyllotoxins (Kane and Gottesman, 1989).

Another drug-resistance gene is the methylguanine methyltransferase gene (*MGMT*) which encodes an enzymatic activity which can repair O6-alkylguanine DNA adducts. These adducts can be induced by a number of different antineoplastic agents, such as BCNU, ACNU, CCNU, dacarbazine, temozolomide, streptozotocin and procarbazine. They are cytotoxic, a property which forms the basis of their nonselective antineoplastic effects. Although there may be several mechanisms for inherent and acquired resistance to these agents, such as high levels of, or the induction of high levels of, glutathione and polyamine, it appears that DNA repair of the adducts is the major form of protection and resistance. The O6-alkylguanine DNA alkyltransferase enzymatic activity encoded by the *MGMT* gene appears to be the predominant gene for the repair of these adducts.

Another drug-resistance gene is the gene encoding dihydrofolate reductase (*DHFR*). *DHFR* catalyzes the NADPH-dependent reduction of folic acid to dihydrofolate. Methotrexate (MTX), a commonly used antineoplastic agent, binds to and inactivates *DHFR*. Two mechanisms for MTX resistance are:

1. acquired mutations in *DHFR* which alter the affinity and binding of MTX;
2. amplification or overexpression of wild-type *DHFR*.

Other genes which may find a role in genetically engineering drug resistance are aldehyde dehydrogenase, and superoxide dismutase.

The major sites of nonspecific, systemic toxicity associated with the current cytotoxic antineoplastic agents are bone marrow, gastrointestinal and respiratory epithelial mucosa, hair follicles, and male reproductive organs. Other drug-specific toxicities are commonly seen as well, such as cardiotoxicity of the anthracyclines and pulmonary toxicities of the nitrosoureas. Transduction of genes into hematopoietic progenitor cells is technically challenging but feasible. At present, there is no technology available to perform effective gene transfer to the 'stem cells' of the dividing epithelial layer in the gastrointestinal and respiratory tracts. This is essential for this technique to be adopted to protect against mucositis. Mucositis may become the major rate-limiting toxicity of conventional antineoplastic drugs due to the fact that autologous bone marrow transplants, growth factors, and other cytokines are becoming very effective at addressing bone marrow toxicites. For drug-resistance gene therapy to have a major impact in the treatment of cancer, there must be significant technical advances in targeted gene delivery.

There are a number of human clinical trials assessing the utility of the *MDR-1* gene as a therapeutic agent (Deisseroth et al., 1994; Hesdorffer et al., 1994; O'Shaughnessy et al., 1994). These trials are designed to evaluate whether bone marrow can be genetically generated which has increased resistance to cytotoxic drugs, enabling higher doses of these drugs to be used. These trials involve patients scheduled for autologous bone marrow transplation.

Other applications of drug-resistance genes

Genetically engineering drug-resistance genes into the bone marrow has applications other than chemotherapy dose escalation. Correction of certain genetic disorders will be dependent upon the transduction and expression of correct genetic information in mature blood cells. Present technology results in very low gene-transfer efficiencies and short-term expression. If a very selective drug-resistance gene was cotransduced with the target gene, then subtle selective pressure could be applied to enrich the bone marrow stem cells which express the target gene.

References

Anderson, W. F. (1984). Prospects for human gene therapy. *Science*, **226**: 401–9.

Austin, E. A. and Huber, B. E. (1993). A first step in the development of gene therapy for colorectal carcinoma: Cloning, sequencing and expression of *E. coli* cytosine deaminase. *Molecular Pharmacology*, **43**: 380–7.

Bertolini, F., de Monte, L., Corsini, C. et al. (1994). Retrovirus-mediated transfer of the multidrug resistance gene into human haematopoietic progenitor cells. *British Journal of Haematology*, **88**: 318–24.

Borrelli, E., Heyman, R., Hsi, M. and Evans, R. M. (1988). Targeting of an inducible toxic phenotype in animal cells. *Proceedings of the National Academy of Sciences of the United States of America*, **85**: 7572–6.

Borrelli, E., Heyman, R. A., Arias, C., Sawchenko, P. E. and Evans, R. M. (1989). Transgenic mice with inducible dwarfism. *Nature*, **339**: 538–41.

Culver, K. W., Ram, Z., Wallbridge, S., Ishii, H., Oldfield, E. H. and Blaese, R. M. (1992). In vivo gene transfer with retroviral vector-producing cells for treatment of experimental brain tumors. *Science*, **256**: 1550–2.

Davidson, R. L., Kaufman, E. R., Crumpacker, C. S. and Schnipper, L. E. (1981). Inhibition of herpes simplex virus transformed and nontransformed cells by acycloguanosine: Mechanisms of uptake and toxicity. *Virology*, 113: 9–19.

Deisseroth, A., Kavanagh, J. and Chaplin, R. (1994). Use of safety-modified retroviruses to introduce chemotherapy resistance sequences into normal hematopoietic cells for chemoprotection during therapy of ovarian cancer: A pilot trial. *Human Gene Therapy*, **5**: 1507–22.

Donahue, R. E., Kessler, S. W., Bodine, D., McDonagh, K., Dinbar, C., Goodman, S., Agricola, B., Byrne, E., Raffeld, M., Moen, R., Bacher, J., Zsebo, K. M. and Niennhuis, A. W. (1993). Helper virus induced T-cells in nonhuman primates after retroviral mediated gene transfer. *Journal of Experimental Medicine*, **176**: 1125–35.

Elion, G. B. (1982). Mechanism of action and selectivity of acyclovir. *The American Journal of Medicine*, **118**: 289–302.

Elion, G. B., Furman, P. A., Fyfe, J. A., De Miranda, P., Beauchamp, L. and Schaefer, H. J. (1978). Thymidine kinase from herpes simplex virus phosphorylates – the new antiviral compound, 9-(2-hydroxyethoxymethyl)guanine. *Proceedings of the National Academy of Sciences of the United States of America*, **74**: 5716–20.

Flasshove, M., Banerjee, D., Mineishi, S. et al. (1995). Ex vivo expansion and selection of human CD+34 peripheral blood progenitor cells after introduction of a mutated dihydrofolate reductase cDNA via retroviral gene transfer. *Blood*, **85**: 566–74.

Furman, P. A., McGuirt, P. V., Keller, P. M., Fyfe, J. A. and Elion, G. B. (1980). Inhibition by acyclovir of cell growth and DNA synthesis of cells biochemically transformed with herpesvirus genetic information. *Virology*, **102**: 420–30.

Fyfe, J. A., Keller, P. M., Furman, P. A., Miller, R. L. and Elion, G. B. (1978). 9-(2-hydroxyethoxymethyl) guanine inhibits herpes simplex virus replication. *Journal of Biological Chemistry*, **253**: 8721–7.

Hesdorffer, C., Antman, K. and Bank, A. (1994). Human MDR gene transfer in patients with advanced cancer. *Human Gene Therapy*, **5**: 1151–60.

Heyman, R. A., Borrelli, E., Lesley, J., Anderson, D., Richman, D. S., Baird, S. M., Hyman, R. and Evans, R. M. (1989). Thymidine kinase obliteration: creation of transgenic mice with controlled immune deficiency. *Proceedings of the National Academy of Sciences of the United States of America*, **86**: 2698–702.

Huber, B. E., Richards, C. A. and Krenitsky, T. A. (1991). Retroviral-mediated gene therapy for the treatment of hepatocellular carcinoma: An innovative approach for cancer therapy. *Proceedings of the National Academy of Sciences of the United States of America*, **88**: 8039–43.

Huber, B. E., Austin, E. A., Good, S. S., Knick, V. C., Tibbels, S. and Richards, C. A. (1993). In vivo activity of 5-Fcyt on human colorectal carcinoma cells genetically modified to express cytosine deaminase. *Cancer Research*, **53**: 4619–26.

Huber, B. E., Austin, E. A., Richards, C. A., Davis, S. T. and Good, S. S. (1994). Metabolism of 5-FCYT to 5-FURa in human colorectal tumor cells transduced with the cytosine deaminase gene: Significant antitumor effects when only a small percentage of tumor cells express cytosine deaminase. *Proceedings of the National Academy of Sciences of the United States of America*, **91**: 8301–6.

Kane, S. and Gottesman, M. (1989). Multidrug resistance in the laboratory and clinic. *Cancer Cells*, **1**: 33–6.

Khil, M. S., Kim, J. K., Mullen, C. A., Kim, S. H. and Freytag, S. O. (1996). Radiosensitization by 5FCyt of human colorectal carcinoma cells in culture transduced with cytosine deaminase gene. *Clinical Cancer Research*, **2**: 53–7.

Kucera, L. S., Furman, P. A. and Elion, G. B. (1983). Inhibition by acyclovir of herpes simplex virus type 2 morphology transformed cell growth in tissue culture and tumor-bearing animals. *Journal of Medical Virology*, **12**: 119–27.

Miller, A. D. (1990). Gene therapy. *Blood*, **76**: 271–8.

Miller, D. G., Adam, M. A. and Miller, A. D. (1990). Gene transfer by retroviral vectors occurs only in cells that are actively replicating at the time of infection. *Molecular and Cellular Biology*, **10**: 4238–42.

Moolten, F. L. (1976). Genetic mosaicism and the control of cancer. *Medical Hypotheses*, **2**: 79–81.

Moolten, F. L. (1990). Mosaicism induced by gene insertion as a means of improving chemotherapeutic selectivity. *Critical Reviews in Immunology*, **10**: 203–33.

Moolten, F. L. and Wells, J. M. (1990). Curability of tumors bearing herpes thymidine kinase genes transferred by retroviral vectors. *Journal of the National Cancer Institute*, **82**: 297–300.

Mullen, C. A., Kilstrup, M. and Blaese, R. M. (1992). Transfer of the bacterial gene for cytosine deaminase to mammalian cells confers lethal sensitivity to 5-Fcyt: a negative selection system. *Proceedings of the National Academy of Sciences of the United States of America*, **89**: 33–7.

Oldfield, E. H., Ram, Z., Culver, K. W., Blaese, R. M. and DeVroom, H. L. (1993). Gene therapy for the treatment of brain tumors using intra-tumoral transduction with the thymidine kinase gene and intravenous ganciclovir. *Human Gene Therapy*, **4**: 39–69.

O'Shaughnessy, J., Cowan, K. and Nienhuis, A. (1994). Retroviral mediated transfer into hematopoietic stem cells during autologous transplantation after intensive chemotherapy for metastatic breast cancer. *Human Gene Therapy*, **5**: 891–911.

Plautz, G., Nabel, E. G. and Nabel, G. J. (1991). Selective elimination of recombinant genes in vivo with a suicide retroviral vector. *New Biology*, **3**: 709–15.

Ross, S. R. and Solter, D. (1985). Glucocorticoid regulation of mouse mammary tumor virus sequences in transgenic mice. *Proceedings of the National Academy of Sciences of the United States of America*, **82**: 5880–4.

St Clair, M. H., Lambe, C. U. and Furman, P. A. (1987). Inhibition by ganciclovir of cell growth and DNA synthesis of cells biochemically transformed with herpesvirus genetic information. *Antimicrobial Agents and Chemotherapy*, **31**: 844–9.

Ward, M., Richardoson, C., Pioli, P. et al. (1994). Transfer and expression of the human multiple drug resistance gene in human CD+34 cells. *Blood*, **84**: 1408–14.

Weichselbaum, R. R., Hallahan, D. H., Sukhatme, V. P. and Kufe, D. W. (1992). Gene therapy targeting by ionizing radiation. *International Journal of Radiation Oncology, Biology Physics*, **24**: 565–7.

5

Oncogene inactivation and replacement strategies for cancer

JACK A. ROTH

The concept of gene replacement for disease logically followed from the observation that certain diseases are caused by the inheritance of a single functionally defective gene. Diseases caused by a known monogenic defect, such as adenosine deaminase deficiency or Gaucher's disease, could be treated and potentially cured by insertion and expression of a normal copy of the mutant or deleted gene in host cells. This can be conceptualized as 'gene replacement therapy' and represents the basic framework for the development of gene therapy approaches to monogenic diseases.

The identification of specific genes that contribute to the development of the cancer cell presents an opportunity to use these genes and their products as prevention and treatment targets. This is a considerably more complex situation than the monogenic diseases as the development of cancer is associated with multiple genetic abnormalities. The gene families implicated in carcinogenesis include dominant oncogenes and tumor suppressor genes (Bishop, 1991; Weinberg, 1992). An example of the diversity of genes implicated in a common cancer, lung cancer, is shown in Table 5.1. Proto-oncogenes (normal genes that are the homologs of oncogenes) participate in critical cell functions, including signal transduction and transcription. Only a single mutant allele is required for malignant transformation. Primary modifications in the dominant oncogenes that confer gain of transforming function include point mutation, amplification, translocation, and rearrangement. Tumor suppressor genes appear to require homozygous loss of function by either mutation or deletion or by a combination of these. Some tumor suppressor genes appear to play a role in the governance of proliferation by regulation of transcription. Alterations in the expression of dominant oncogenes and tumor suppressor genes may influence certain characteristics of cells that contribute to the malignant phenotype.

Many genetic abnormalities are present in cancer cell lines and fresh tumor

Table 5.1. *Oncogenes and Tumor Suppressor Genes Altered in Lung Cancer*

SCLC	NSCLC
Oncogenes	
c-myc*	K-ras*
L-myc	N-ras
N-myc	H-ras
c-raf	c-myc
c-myb	c-raf
c-erbB-1 (EGF-R)	c-fur*
c-fms	c-fes
c-rlf	c-erbB-1 (EGF-R)
	c-erbB-2 (Her2, neu)
	c-sis
	bcl-1
Tumor suppressor genes	
p53*	p53*
RB*	RB

*Most frequently altered genes in tumors or cell lines evaluated.
From Greenblott, M. S., Reddel, R. R. and Harris, C. C.
Carcinogenesis, cellular, and molecular biology of lung cancer. In
J. A. Roth, J. C. Ruckdeschel and T. H. Weisenberger (eds.)
Thoracic Oncology, 2nd edition, New York: W. B. Saunders
Company. In press.

samples (Yokota et al., 1987; Ibson et al., 1987; Vogelstein et al., 1988, 1989). This is evident at the chromosomal level, where multiple abnormalities have been identified. The numbers of identified oncogenes and tumor suppressor genes have been growing. Although it was believed at one time that gene replacement therapy would not be possible in cancer because of the difficulties associated with correcting multiple genetic abnormalities in one cell, several observations suggest that gene replacement in cancer is feasible.

Several studies have shown that correction of a single genetic defect, for example, eliminating expression of a dominant oncogene or adding a normal copy of a tumor suppressor gene to a cell with deleted or mutated copies, reduced or eliminated critical characteristics of the malignant phenotype such as tumorigenicity or anchorage-independent growth (Bookstein et al., 1990; Mukhopadhyay et al., 1991; Takahasti et al., 1992). The studies done in our laboratory that support this concept, and their application to animal models and clinical protocols, are described later in this chapter.

Efficient delivery of the therapeutic gene to the cancer cell is essential to mediate a therapeutic effect. It was previously believed that most available delivery system vectors were very inefficient in transducing cancer cells. Because selectivity of proviral integration for proliferating cells favors infection of tumor cells, viruses were among the earliest delivery systems used, particularly the retroviruses. Fresh human cancers have a relatively high fraction of proliferating tumor cells (Kitamura et al., 1995; Tamiya et al., 1995; Knol et al., 1995). Retroviruses have been extensively studied as delivery vehicles in gene-transfer protocols (Danos and Mulligan, 1988). Retroviral vectors have been created that lack genes essential for replication. The replication-defective vectors are capable of infecting cells and integrating as a provirus, which will then express recombinant genes. Studies in models of human tumors in-vitro and in *nu/nu* mice have shown that uptake of a retroviral vector is efficient enough to mediate a therapeutic effect (Zhang et al., 1993, 1994; Georges et al., 1993; Fujiwara et al., 1994a). Because retroviruses are integrated and express the transgene primarily in proliferating cells, retroviral vectors may be selective for cancer cells. Adenoviral vectors will be taken up by both dividing and nondividing cells. Even a single infection of an adenoviral vector in culture is sufficient to infect more than 90% of cancer cells (Zhang et al., 1994). Furthermore, viral vectors are able to penetrate three-dimensional tumor cell matrices (Fujiwara et al., 1993).

Despite the relatively high efficiencies of cancer cell transduction achieved by viral vectors, it is doubtful that every cancer cell can be transduced. Transduced cells can cause the death of nontransduced cells by mediating a 'bystander effect.' This effect was first noted in brain tumor cells transduced with the herpes simplex thymidine kinase gene and then exposed to gancyclovir (Culver et al., 1992). It may be mediated by toxic metabolites of gancyclovir being passed through gap junctions, by phagocytosis of apoptotic vesicles, or by immunologic responses (Freeman et al., 1993; Bi et al., 1993; Vile et al., 1994). The bystander effect has also been observed in lung cancer cells with endogenous mutant *p53* that has been transduced with a retrovirus expressing the wild-type *p53*, although a different mechanism is probably involved (Cai et al., 1993). These observations suggest that gene replacement in cancer has potential for mediating therapeutic effects. Given the multiple genetic lesions in cancer cells, a critical question will be which genes to target. The most promising are dominant oncogenes and tumor suppressor genes.

Dominant oncogenes

The *ras* family of oncogenes (homologous to the rat sarcoma virus) has three primary members (H-*ras* , K-*ras*, and N-*ras*), which are among the most common activated oncogenes found in human cancer (Bos, 1989). The *ras* genes code for a protein (p21) which is located on the inner surface of the plasma membrane, has GTPase activity, and may participate in signal transduction. The *ras* oncogenes are activated by point nucleotide mutations that alter the amino acid sequence of p21.

In our laboratory, antisense technology was used to examine the effects of eliminating expression of a mutant K-*ras* oncogene in lung cancer cells (Mukhopadhyay et al., 1991). A homozygous mutation at codon 61 was detected in the NCI-H460a large cell undifferentiated non-small cell lung cancer (NSCLC) cell line clone, which has a normal glutamine residue (CAA) substituted by histidine (CAT). An antisense K-*ras* RNA construct was developed which selectively blocked the production of mutant K-*ras* RNA and reduced the growth rate of H460a tumors in *nu/nu* mice. Although cancer cells have multiple genetic abnormalities, the reversal of a single abnormality appears to have profound effects on fundamental properties of the malignant phenotype, such as rapid proliferation and tumorigenicity. This was observed when the antisense K-*ras* plasmid expression vector was transfected into H460a cells which have, in addition to a K-*ras* mutation, five chromosomal deletions (chromosomes 1, 2, 9, 12, 16).

Because retroviruses and cells modified by retroviral transduction have little acute toxicity, multiple treatments with high-titer preparations are feasible. The retroviral vector system developed to efficiently transduce a K-*ras* antisense construct into human cancer cells contained a 1.8 kb K-*ras* gene fragment DNA in antisense orientation to a β-actin promoter inserted into retroviral vector LNSX (Zhang et al., 1993). Colony formation in soft agarose and tumorigenicity in an orthotopic *nu/nu* mouse model by H460a cells transduced by this vector, which expressed antisense K-*ras*, were dramatically decreased (Georges et al., 1993). We conclude that an antisense construct for K-*ras* can be expressed effectively in a retroviral vector that can efficiently transduce human cancer cells. These studies show that retroviral supernatants expressing the appropriate therapeutic construct can mediate antitumor effects; that an antisense construct can mediate therapeutic tumor regression in vivo; and that antitumor effects can occur as a result of inhibition of oncogene expression.

Tumor suppressor genes

The *p53* gene encodes a 393-amino-acid phosphoprotein, also called p53, that can form complexes with viral proteins such as large-T antigen and E1B and is the most commonly mutated gene identified to date in human cancers (Hollstein et al., 1991). Missense mutations are common in the *p53* gene and in many cases will functionally impair the *p53* gene product (Raycroft, Wu and Lozano, 1990; Fields and Jang, 1990). The mechanism of *p53* transformation may vary depending on the type of *p53* mutation. The *p53* gene appears multifunctional, with major domains that can transactivate, bind proteins, bind sequence-specific DNA, and oligomerize with *p53*. Abnormalities in one or more of these functions could eliminate or reduce the tumor suppressor function of *p53*. Failure of the mutant *p53* to activate transcription of molecules essential for regulating the cell cycle and DNA repair, or the untimely expression of molecules transcriptionally enhanced by the mutant *p53*, may make the cell more susceptible to genetic instability. Certain mutations also have a dominant transforming capability. The wild-type *p53* gene may suppress genes that contribute to uncontrolled cell growth and proliferation or activate genes that suppress uncontrolled cell growth. Thus, absence or inactivation of wild-type *p53* may contribute to transformation. The *p53* gene also regulates cell cycle progression. If DNA damage occurs, the cell will arrest at the G-1 checkpoint until the damage is repaired. Failure to repair DNA damage may then trigger apoptosis (programmed cell death).

A retroviral vector-mediated system was established to allow efficient transduction of the wild-type *p53* gene into human lung cancer cell lines H358a (deleted *p53*) and H322a (mutant *p53*) (Cai et al., 1993). LNSX/*p53* constructs incorporating *p53* cDNA driven by a β-actin promoter mediated stable integration of *p53*. *p53* mRNA and protein were detected in these cell lines six months after transduction by northern and western blot analyses. Restoration of the wild-type *p53* gene suppressed growth in the two transduced cell lines but had no effect in another transduced tumor cell line, H460a, which has an endogenous wild-type *p53* gene. Mixing experiments showed that transduced cells could reduce the growth rate of nontransduced cells, indicating a bystander effect. This reduction may have been mediated by factors shed into the supernatant of the transduced cell cultures.

Mutations in the *p53* tumor suppressor gene are common in human lung cancers. The wild-type form of *p53* is dominant over the mutant, and thus restoration of wild-type *p53* function in lung cancer cells may suppress their growth as tumors. We investigaged the therapeutic efficacy of direct administration of a retroviral wild-type *p53* (wt-*p53*) expression vector (LN*p53*B) in an orthotopic human lung cancer model (Fujiwara et al., 1994a). Thirty days after tumor cell inoculation, 63–80% of the control mice showed macroscopic tumors of the right mainstream bronchus. LN*p53*B suppressed H226Br tumor formation in 62–100% of mice, and the effect was dose dependent. These results suggest that direct administration of a retroviral vector expressing wt-*p53* may inhibit local growth in-vivo of human lung cancer cells with abnormal *p53* expression. We conclude that development of gene-replacement treatment strategies based on the type of mutations found in target cancers is warranted, and may lead to the development of new adjunctive therapies and gene-specific prevention strategies for lung cancer.

Adenoviral vectors can transduce both dividing and nondividing cells and may have tropism for lung epithelium. We developed an adenoviral vector for delivery of wild-type *p53*. The *p53* expression cassette, which contains human cytomegalovirus promoter, wild-type *p53* cDNA, and SV40 early polyadenylation signal, was inserted between the Xba 1 and Cla 1 sites of plasmid pXCJL.1 (a gift from Dr F. L. Graham). The *p53* shuttle vector (pEC53) and the recombinant plasmid pJM17 (Mcgrory, Bautista and Graham, 1988) were cotransfected into 293 cells (Graham and Eb, 1973) by liposome-mediated transfection with DOTAP. A high level of expression of exogenous *p53* was achieved in H358 cells that were infected by Ad5CMV-*p53* at a multiplicity of infection (MOI) of 30 plaque-forming units (PFU)/cell. When H322 or H460 cells were infected at the same MOI, the level of expression of the exogenous *p53* gene was three times higher than that of the endogenous mutated protein in H322, and 14 times higher than that of the endogenous wild-type protein in H460 cells.

The time course of the expression of the exogenous *p53* after a single infection of 10 PFU/cell was studied in H358 cells. The protein expression peaked at postinfection day 3, sharply decreased after day 5, and lasted for at least 15 days. This is a critical point with respect to safety of the vector. Transient *p53* expression is sufficient for mediating apoptosis. If normal cells take up the vector, they will express the exogenous *p53* for only a short time and their growth will be unaffected. Ad5CMV-*p53* inhibited the proliferation of lung cancer cells with mutated or deleted *p53*, but only minimally affected the growth of cells with wild-type *p53*. The efficacy of Ad5CMV-*p53* in inhibiting tumorigenicty was evaluated in the mouse model of orthotopic human lung cancer (Georges et al., 1993). H226Br cells which originated from a squamous lung cancer that metastasized to brain and have a point mutation (ATC to GTC) at exon 7, codon 254, of the *p53* gene were used to induce tumors. After six weeks, only 25% of the Ad5CMV-*p53*-treated mice formed tumors, whereas in the control groups 70–80% of the treated mice formed tumors. The average tumor size of the Ad5CMV-*p53* group was significantly smaller than those of the control groups. These results indicate that Ad5CMV-*p53* can prevent H226Br from forming tumors in the mouse model of orthotopic human lung cancer.

We examined whether Ad-*p53* and cisplatin (CDDP) given in a sequential combination could induce synergistic tumor regression in vivo (Fujiwara et al., 1994b). Following three daily direct intratumoral injections of Ad-*p53*, H358a tumors subcutaneously transplanted in *nu/nu* mice showed a modest slowing of growth; Ad-*p53*-injected tumors, however, regressed if CDDP was administered intraperitoneally for three days. Histologic examination revealed necrosis of tumor tissue in the area where Ad-*p53* was injected in mice treated with CDDP. In-situ staining showed extensive areas of apoptosis. In contrast, tumors treated with CDDP alone or AD-*p53* alone showed no apoptosis.

Clinical applications

These studies provide a rationale for novel clinical protocols recently approved by the National Institutes of Health (NIH) Recombinant DNA Advisory Committee (RAC) and US Food and Drug Administation (FDA) to inhibit expression of mutant K-*ras* p21 or replace a defective *p53* gene with intratumoral injection of recombinant retrovirus expressing antisense K-*ras* or normal *p53*, respectively. Patients whose bronchus is blocked with unresectable lung cancer which has a *p53* mutation will have the tumor that remains after endoscopic resection directly injected with the appropriate retroviral supernatant. Patients with unresectable local tumors or isolated metastases may undergo radiologic image-guided injection of the vector. Toxicity, integration of the proviral DNA by tumor cells, and rate of tumor regrowth will be monitored.

A second protocol, which has also received NIH RAC and FDA approval, will test the adenovirus-*p53* vector (Ad5CMV-*p53*). Patients for this protocol must have either an endobronchial tumor accessible by the bronchoscope, with some clinical evidence of bronchial obstruction, or advanced local–regional lung cancer which is unresectable. The study will be an open-label upward dose-ranging trial of the vector and will be done in two phases. It is not known what toxic effects, if any, will be caused by the adenovirus. The first phase of the study will allow assessment of toxic effects related only to the vector. Patients will receive one intratumoral or intrapleural injection of Ad5CMV-*p53*. The initial dose will be 10^6 PFU.

Following completion of this phase, a second phase will evaluate Ad5CMV-*p53* plus CDDP administered concurrently based on evidence of synergy between wild-type *p53* and CDDP (Fujiwara et al., 1994b). Patients in this group will receive one intratumoral injection of Ad5CMV-*p53* with concurrent CDDP (30 mg/m^2), with two additional doses of CDDP on days 2 and 3. Three patients will be entered at each dose level, with six patients entered at the maximum tolerated or maximum attainable dose (limitation imposed by production of the adenovirus). The adenovirus dose will increase in log$_{10}$ increments for each group. The objectives of the trial are to determine the maximum tolerated dose of the wild-type *p53* adenoviral vector given with and without CDDP in patients with refractory lung cancer to determine the qualitative and quantitative toxicity and reversibility of toxicity of this treatment approach; and to document observed antitumor activity of this treatment approach.

A third RAC-approved and FDA-approved protocol will attempt to prevent local recurrences in patients with resectable recurrent head and neck cancers by treatment of the incision site with Ad5CMV-*p53*. Patients with unresectable lung cancer obstructing a bronchus or advanced regional tumor which has a K-*ras* or *p53* mutation will have the tumor directly injected either bronchoscopically or percutaneously under radiologic guidance with the appropriate retroviral supernatant. Toxicity, integration of the proviral DNA by tumor cells, and rate of tumor regrowth will be monitored.

Successful therapy and prevention interventions that reverse genetic lesions may be possible. Genetic constructs could specifically inhibit expression of mutant proteins by dominant oncogenes and could replace the function of deleted or mutated tumor suppressor genes if they could be delivered with high efficiency to tumor cells in vivo. Viral vectors have this potential. The aerodigestive tract is suited to this approach because high concentrations of these relatively nontoxic agents could be achieved with local installation, thus avoiding the dilutional effects of intravenous injection. For example, restoration of normal *p53* function in the tumor may increase radiosensitivity (Lee and Bernstein, 1993; Pardo et al., 1994).

Intervention to halt the progression of premalignant lesions to invasive cancer may be possible. Premalignant lesions such as bronchial dysplasia or Barrett's epithelium have tumor suppressor gene mutations (Casson et al., 1991; Bennett et al., 1993). Preventing the development of invasive cancers would clearly be preferable to treating established cancer. However, there is also a potential role for these agents in the treatment of patients with more advanced cancer. Local recurrence or persistence of local disease is still a major problem for many cancers such as lung, head and neck, and pancreas. Intralesional injections or adjuvant use of gene constructs to prevent local recurrence after surgery could be considered. Limited metastatic disease could be injected with these agents percutaneously. If these agents are efficacious, their lack of toxicity may provide a sufficiently high therapeutic index for them to be used as an adjuvant to surgery to treat patients with earlier stages of cancer, or as prevention for second primary cancers for individuals with genetic abnormalities in premalignant lesions. The high titers achievable with adenoviral vectors suggest that they could be used systemically. Vector targeting by expression of receptor ligands in the viral capsid is also possible. Although much research needs to be done, the possibility of specific gene targeting with a high therapeutic index makes this a potentially promising area for investigation.

References

Bennett, W. P., Colby, T. V., Travis, W. D. et al. (1993). p53 protein accumulates frequently in early bronchial neoplasia. *Cancer Research*, **53**: 4817–22.

Bi, W. L., Parysek, L. M., Warnick, R. and Stambrook, P. J. (1993). In vitro evidence that metabolic cooperation is responsible for the bystander effect observed with HSV tk retroviral gene therapy. *Human Gene Therapy*, **4**: 725–31.

Bishop, J. M. (1991). Molecular themes in oncogenesis. *Cell*, **64**: 235–48.

Bookstein, R., Shew, J. Y., Chen, P. L., Scully, P. and Lee, W. H. (1990). Suppression of tumorigenicity of human prostate carcinoma cells by replacing a mutated RB gene. *Science*, **247**: 712–15.

Bos, J. I. (1989). ras oncogenes in human cancer: a review. *Cancer Research*, **49**: 4682–9.

Cai, D. W., Mukhopadhyay, T., Liu, Y. J., Fujiwara, T. and Roth, J. A. (1993). Stable expression of the wild-type p53 gene in human lung cancer cells after retrovirus-mediated gene transfer. *Human Gene Therapy*, **4**: 617–24.

Casson, A. G., Mukhopadhyay, T., Cleary, K. R., Ro, J. Y., Levin, B. and Roth, J. A. (1991). p53 gene mutations in Barrett's epithelium and esophageal cancer. *Cancer Research*, **51**: 4495–9.

Culver, K. W., Ram, Z., Wallbridge, S., Ishii, H., Oldfield, E. H. and Blaese, R. M. (1992). In vivo gene transfer with retroviral vector-producer cells for treatment of experimental brain tumors. *Science*, **256**: 1550–2.

Danos, O. and Mulligan, R. C. (1988). Safe and efficient generation of recombinant retroviruses with amphotropic and ecotropic host ranges. *Proceedings of the National Academy of Sciences of the United States of America*, **85**: 6460–4.

Fields, S. and Jang, S. K. (1990). Presence of a potent transcription activating sequence in the p53 protein. *Science*, **249**: 1046–51.

Freeman, S. M., Abboud, C. N., Whartenby, K. A., Packman, C. H., Koeplin, D. S., Moolten, F. L. and Abraham, G. N. (1993). The 'bystander effect': Tumor regression when a fraction of the tumor mass is genetically modified. *Cancer Research*, **53**: 5274–82.

Fujiwara, T., Cai, D. W., Georges, R. N., Mukhopadhyay, T., Grimm, E. A. and Roth, J. A. (1994a). Therapeutic effect of a retroviral wild-type p53 expression vector in an orthotopic lung cancer model. *Journal of the National Cancer Institute*, **86**: 1458–62.

Fujiwara, T., Grimm, E. A., Mukhopadhyay, T., Cai, D. W., Owen-Schaub, L. B. and Roth, J. A. (1993). A retroviral wild-type p53 expression vector penetrates human lung cancer spheroids and inhibits growth by inducing apoptosis. *Cancer Research*, **53**: 4129–33.

Fujiwara, T., Grimm, E. A., Mukhopadhyay, T., Zhang, W. W., Owen-Schaub, L. B. and Roth, J. A. (1994b). Induction of chemosensitivity in human lung cancer cells in vivo by adenoviral-mediated transfer of the wild-type p53 gene. *Cancer Research*, **54**: 2287–91.

Georges, R. N., Mukhopadhyay, T., Zhang, Y. J., Yen, N. and Roth, J. A. (1993). Prevention of orthotopic human lung cancer growth by intratracheal instillation of a retroviral antisense K-*ras* construct. *Cancer Research*, **53**: 1743–6.

Graham, F. L. and Eb, V. D. (1973). A new technique for the assay of infectivity of human adenovirus 5 DNA. *Virology*, **52**: 456–67.

Greenblott, M. S., Reddel, R. R. and Harris, C. C. (1995). Carcinogenesis, cellular, and molecular biology of lung cancer. In J. A. Roth, J. C. Ruckdeschel and T. H. Weisenberger (eds.) *Thoracic Oncology*, pp. 5–22. W. B. Saunders, New York.

Hollstein, M., Sidransky, D., Vogelstein, B. and Harris, C. C. (1991). p53 mutations in human cancers. *Science*, **352**: 49–53.

Ibson, J. M., Waters, J. J., Twentyman, P. R., Bleehen, N. M. and Rabbitts, P. H. (1987). Oncogene amplification and chromosomal abnormalities in small cell lung cancer. *Journal of Cell Biochemistry*, **33**: 267–88.

Kitamura, H., Kameda, Y., Nakamura, N. et al. (1995). Proliferative potential and p53 overexpression in precursor and early stage lesions of bronchioloalveolar lung carcinoma. *American Journal of Pathology*, **146**: 876–87.

Knol, J. A., Walker, S. C., Robertson, J. M. et al. (1995). Incorporation of 5-bromo-2'-deoxyuridine into colorectal liver metastases and liver in patients receiving a 7-day hepatic arterial infusion. *Cancer Research*, **55**: 3687–91.

Lee, J. M. and Bernstein, A. (1993). p53 mutations increase resistance to ionizing radiation. *Proceedings of the National Academy of Sciences of the United States of America*, **90**: 5742–6.

Mcgrory, W. J., Bautista, D. S. and Graham, F. L. (1988). A simple technique for the rescue of early region 1 mutations into infectious human adenovirus type 5. *Virology*, **163**: 614–17.

Mukhopadhyay, T., Tainsky, M., Cavender, A. C. and Roth, J. A. (1991). Specific inhibition of K-*ras* expression and tumorigenicity of lung cancer cells by antisense RNA. *Cancer Research*, **51**: 1744–8.

Pardo, F. S., Su, M., Borek, C., Preffer, F., Dombkowski, D., Gerweck, L. and Schmidt, E. V. (1994). Transfection of rat embryo cells with mutant p53 increases the intrinsic radiation resistance. *Radiation Research*, **140**: 180–5.

Raycroft, L., Wu, H. and Lozano, G. (1990). Transcriptional activation by wild-type but not transforming mutants of the p53 anti-oncogene. *Science*, **249**: 1049–51.

Takahashi, T., Carbone, D., Nau, M. M., Hida, T., Linnoila, I., Ueda, R. and Minna, J. D. (1992). Wild-type but not mutant p53 suppresses the growth of human lung cancer cells bearing multiple genetic lesions. *Cancer Research*, **52**: 2340–3.

Tamiya, T., Wei, M. X., Chase, M., Ono, Y., Lee, F., Breakefield, X. O. and Chiocca, E. A. (1995). Transgene inheritance and retroviral infection contribute to the efficiency of gene expression in solid tumors inoculated with retroviral vector producer cells. *Gene Therapy*, **2**: 531–8.

Vile, R. G., Nelson, J. A., Castleden, S., Chong, H. and Hart, I. R. (1994). Systemic gene therapy of murine melanoma using tissue specific expression of the HSVtk gene involves an immune component. *Cancer Research*, **54**: 6228–34.

Vogelstein, B., Fearon, E. R., Hamilton, S. R. et al. (1988). Genetic alterations during colorectal-tumor development. *New England Journal of Medicine*, **319**: 525–32.

Vogelstein, B., Fearon, E. R., Kern, S. E. et al. (1989). Allelotype of colorectal carcinomas. *Science*, **224**: 207–11.

Weinberg, R. A. (1992). Tumor suppressor genes. *Science*, **254**: 1138–45.

Yokota, J., Wada, M., Shimosato, Y., Terada, M. and Sugimura, T. (1987). Loss of heterozygosity on chromosomes 3, 13, and 17 in small-cell carcinoma and on chromosome 3 in adenocarcinoma of the lung. *Proceedings of the National Academy of Sciences of the United States of America*, **84**: 9252–6.

Zhang, Y. J., Mukhopadhyay, T., Donehower, L. W., Georges, R. N. and Roth, J. A. (1993). Retroviral vector-mediated transduction of K-*ras* antisense RNA into human lung cancer cells inhibits expression of the malignant phenotype. *Human Gene Therapy*, **4**: 451–60.

Zhang, W. W., Fang, X., Mazur, W., French, B. A., Georges, R. N. and Roth, J. A. (1994). High-efficiency gene transfer and high-level expression of wild-type p53 in human lung cancer cells mediated by recombinant adenovirus. *Cancer Gene Therapy*, **1**: 5–13.

Studies described in this chapter were partially supported by a grant from the National Cancer Institute, National Institutes of Health (RO1 CA45187); by a National Cancer Institute Training Grant (CA09611); by gifts to the Division of Surgery from Tenneco and Exxon for the Core Lab Facility; by the M. D. Anderson Cancer Center Support Core Grant (CA16672); by a grant from the Mathers Foundation; and by a sponsored research agreement with Introgen Therapeutics, Inc.

6

Genetically modified tumor cells as tumor vaccines

JOHN C. KRAUSS, SUYU SHU AND ALFRED E. CHANG

Introduction

Recombinant DNA technology has allowed for the efficient introduction of defined genes into mammalian cells. Utilizing this technology, it has been feasible to express a variety of immunoregulatory proteins in tumor cells in order to modulate the host's immune response to native tumor antigens. The components of the immune response necessary to generate immunity to tumors consist of: (a) emigration of inflammatory cells to the site of tumor growth; (b) processing of tumor antigens by antigen-presenting cells; (c) sensitization of lymphoid cells; and (d) amplification and/or suppression of mature effector cells. Thus, there is a variety of avenues to modulate an immune response by specifically adding defined immune regulatory genes in this process.

Transplantable animal tumors have provided a wealth of information concerning the host antitumor immune response. Depending upon the inherent immunogenicity of the tumor, experimental methods are capable of eliciting systemic immunity to a variety of tumors in naive hosts. Many of the initial studies with genetically modified tumor cells have focused on the ability of the host to reject an inoculum of modified tumor cells, with the induction of systemic immunity to a subsequent challenge of the parental tumor. Hence, the inherent immunogenicity of the tumor being examined is important in interpreting the significance of genetic modification. Tumor immunogenicity has been traditionally defined by transplantation procedures. Table 6.1 presents the framework for discussing immunogenicity that is utilized in this chapter and is based on the ability to immunize animals to resist tumor challenge by various manipulations. The most easily defined tumors are those belonging to the category 'highly immunogenic,' which after inoculation grow and then regress, leaving the animal immune to further challenges with the same tumor. 'Immunogenic' tumors are those that grow progressively in

Table 6.1. *Immunogenicity of transplantable animal tumors*

Designation	Growth characteristics	Method to generate immunity
1. Highly immunogenic	Grows then regresses	Inoculation of tumor cells
2. Immunogenic	Grows progressively	Inoculation of irradiated cells or surgical excision after inoculation
3. Weakly immunogenic	Grows progressively	Inoculation with irradiated cells and adjuvant
4. Poorly or nonimmunogenic	Grows progressively	Inability to generate systemic immunity

normal animals but are capable of inducing systemic immunity by methods such as inoculation with irradiated cells, or allowing the tumor to grow followed by surgical excision. 'Weakly immunogenic' tumors are those that require an immune adjuvant in addition to an inoculum of tumor cells to immunize animals. On the extreme end of the spectrum, 'nonimmunogenic or poorly immunogenic' tumors resist all attempts to generate immunity in animals. It has been postulated that most human tumors are poorly immuno-genic, based on theoretic considerations, and on their spontaneous origins. Strategies to augment antitumor immunity that have the most potential in the development of clinical therapy are those that address the problems associated with poorly immunogenic tumors. However, using immunogenic tumors for experimentation may provide insights into the mechanisms of T cell responses to tumor antigens and of tumor eradication.

Based on theoretical considerations and the results of animal studies, geneti-cally modified tumor cell vaccines are now entering human clinical trials. This chapter addresses selected animal studies upon which these clinical trials are based. The complexity of the immune response to tumor necessitates in-vivo demonstration of antitumor efficacy as the gold standard. Attention is paid to studies in which attempts were made to assess accurately the in-vivo immune-modulating effects of vaccinations with genetically modified tumor cells.

Modulation of major histocompatibility complex molecules

Major histocompatibility complex (MHC) molecules are receptors for peptide antigens and act to 'restrict' immunological responses mediated by specific T cell subsets. There are two types of MHC molecules, Class I and II, which noncovalently complex with antigenic peptides and simultaneously serve as ligands for two subsets of T cells. Class I molecules serve as antigen receptors for CD8 lymphocytes, while Class II molecules perform the same function for CD4 lymphocytes. Some CD8 cells are functionally termed cytotoxic T lymphocytes (CTL) because they are capable of directly killing target cells. CD4 cells are also called helper T cells and respond to antigen stimulation by secreting interleukin 2 (IL-2) as well as many other immunologically active cytokines. Tumor cells have variable expression of MHC molecules, and their relative loss of expression has been postulated to be associated with decreased immunogenicity. Several investigations have focused on upregulating Class I or II MHC expression on tumor cells in order to enhance the host immune response.

Class I MHC molecules

Initial studies by several groups of investigators demonstrated that both chemically induced and virally induced tumors could be rendered less tumorigenic by transfection of syngeneic Class I molecules (Hui, Grosveld and Festenstein, 1984; Wallich et al., 1985; Tanaka et al., 1985). Generally this was manifested by a delayed growth curve of the transfected Class I-expressing cells as compared to control transfected cells. This delayed growth pattern was most apparent at threshold tumorigenic cell doses, and disappeared at higher cell doses. Evidence for a host immune response to the newly introduced Class I protein was demonstrated either by abrogation of decreased tumorigenicity in irradiated hosts, or by abrogation with blocking Class I monoclonal antibodies administered to animals. One study demonstrated the development of systemic immunity in animals that rejected tumors transfected with Class I molecules when rechallenged with the wild-type tumor (Hui et al., 1984).

In 1988, the transfection of Class I genes into tumors was extended to the poorly immunogenic BL6 melanoma, a subline of the spontaneously arisen B16 tumor (Tanaka et al., 1988). The BL6 tumor does not express Class I molecules and is syngeneic to C57BL/6 mice of H-2^b background. Transfection of BL6 cells with the native *H-2K^b* gene reduced tumor growth rates at several tumorigenic doses. Furthermore, immunization with Class I-expressing BL6 cells was able to protect a substantial fraction of mice from a subsequent challenge of the parental tumor in a dose-dependent fashion. In a parallel series of experiments reported in the same study, transfection of allogeneic Class II MHC genes (α and β chains) into BL6 cells did not generate immunity in animals.

Expression of allogeneic Class I molecules can potentially induce an allogeneic rejection response which may modulate the host response to native tumor antigens. Cole et al. reported the results of transfecting an allogeneic *H-2K^b* gene into the *H-2K^k*-expressing SaI fibrosarcoma (Cole et al., 1987). They demonstrated that *H-2K^b* could be expressed on the cell surface of SaI tumor cells. However, the *H-2K^b*-positive tumor cell clones exhibited decreased levels of expression of the endogenous *H-2K^k*. The majority of the *H-2K^b*-expressing clones were not rejected in the syngeneic host, and grew progressively. Furthermore, expression of the *H-2K^b* did not make the cells more susceptible to lysis by CTL or to lectin-dependent cellular cytolysis.

Recent studies reported by Plautz et al. have focused on the expression of allogeneic Class I molecules introduced in vivo to delay or prevent tumor outgrowth (Plautz et al., 1993). When H-2K^b animals (C57Bl/6) were pre-immunized with H-2K^s cells, a weakly immunogenic syngeneic tumor (MCA 106) that was transfected in vivo with the *H-2K^s* gene failed to grow. Gene transfer was accomplished by direct intratumoral inoculation of DNA complexed with liposomes. In this study, the in-vivo gene transfer of an allogeneic MHC Class I gene resulted in prolongation of survival. This effect was presumably T cell dependent, since it was not observed in nude mice. Furthermore, the antitumor effect was not observed in mice treated with DNA encoding for an in-frame deletion mutant of the Class I H-2K^s molecule. Host immunity was demonstrated in the spleens of animals treated by *H-2K^s* gene transfer by the retrieval of cytolytic T cells reactive to parental, unmodified tumor cells.

The results observed in the latter studies have led to the institution of a Phase I/II clinical trial of in-vivo allogeneic MHC Class I gene transfer at the University of Michigan (Nabel et al., 1993). This study was the first to attempt in-vivo gene therapy in humans. It involved five patients with melanoma who were administered liposomes complexed with DNA encoding the human MHC Class I molecule, HLA-B7. The liposome/DNA complexes were injected directly into subcutaneous tumor nodules. All patients were HLA-B7 negative, so they had the potential to mount an allogeneic response directed against the gene product. No evidence of toxicity was noted in the first five patients treated. The presence of plasmid DNA at the tumor site was observed in four of the five patients one week after injection, and evidence of in-vivo transcription was noted in those same patients. Analysis for HLA-B7 protein expression with monoclonal antibodies revealed that about 1% of the tumor cells at the injection site expressed the gene. One patient demonstrated a clinical response of injected and distant tumor nodules, although not all sites of metastatic disease responded. A second trial, using an expression vector for the HLA-B7 allele in combination with β2-microglobulin and an improved formulation of liposomes, is currently being performed.

While the first reported trial of direct injection of DNA into tumors is encouraging, the consistent ability to treat disseminated malignancy in animals or in humans with Class I-transfected tumors has yet to be established. Class I expression appears to increase the immunogenicity of some tumors but not of others in animal models. The problem is exponentially more complex in humans because Class I alleles are defined using serologic methods. Genotypic methods, just being developed, may provide some insight into tumor-prone or tumor-resistant Class I alleles, but the extreme allelic diversity of humans at the MHC locus will almost certainly complicate this analysis. Further understanding of the biology of human Class I genotypes may provide some insights to possible methods to treat tumors with Class I transfection.

Class II MHC molecules

Class II MHC proteins are classically thought to present exogenously synthesized peptides to immune effector cells. Transfection of tumor cells with Class II molecules could potentially enable the tumor to present its own mutated proteins to helper T cells to generate an effective immune response. Depending upon the tumor model, conflicting observations have been reported regarding the immunobiologic effects of transfecting tumors with MHC Class II genes.

Over the last several years, Ostrand-Rosenberg and co-workers have demonstrated that transfection of functional, syngeneic Class II α and β chains increases the immunogenicity of tumors (Ostrand-Rosenberg, Thakur and Clements, 1990; Ostrand-Rosenberg, Roby and Clements, 1991; Clements et al., 1992). It was found that transfection of the Ia^k gene into the Ia^k-negative SaI fibrosarcoma rendered the cells nontumorigenic (Ostrand-Rosenberg et al., 1990). Expression of the Class II gene by the transfectants did not alter the expression of endogenous Class I genes. Animals that rejected the transfected tumors were immune to a challenge with parental tumor. In a subsequent report, these investigators generated tumor transfectants with antigen-presentation-defective cytoplasmic deletion mutants of Class II (Ostrand-Rosenberg et al., 1991). The antigen-presentation-defective mutants retained their tumorigenicity, suggesting that tumor antigen presentation by the intact MHC Class II was a potential mechanism of decreased tumorigenicity. Alternatively, the cytoplasmic deletion mutants could have failed to activate the cell as the wild-type Class II might have done, potentially implicating other mechanisms of reduced tumorigenicity.

These results contrast with the study of Tanaka et al., where Class II transfection did not alter tumorigenicity (Tanaka et al., 1988). These investigators transfected an allogeneic Ia^k gene into the poorly immunogenic BL6 melanoma which is derived from Ia^b-positive mice. The Ia^k gene did not alter the tumorigenicity of the cells in C3H × B6 F1 mice (heterozygous for Ia^k). Furthermore, inoculation of Ia^k-positive cells into the footpad followed by amputation and challenge with parental cells did not afford any immune protection. Expression of the syngeneic Ia^b gene would have made the results more directly comparable to the other reports. However, these results indicated that Class II gene transfection did not generate tumors which were more immunogenic than parental tumor. The presence of other accessory molecules may prove essential to the enhanced immunogenicity of Class II transfectants (see below). Furthermore, the ability of Class II transfected tumors to treat established malignancy needs to be investigated.

Cytokine gene transfection

Engineering tumor cells to secrete cytokines in the microenvironment can potentially augment several phases of the host antitumor immune response. Theoretically, cytokine secretion by tumor cells could: (a) increase the recruitment of antigen-presenting cells in the tumor; (b) promote the proliferation of immune cells; (c) upregulate the expression of molecules on tumor cells necessary for recognition by antigen-presenting cells and/or immune effector cells; and (d) enhance the infiltration of the tumor by immune effector cells. From the plethora of reported studies, there is a strong correlation between the amount of cytokine secreted and the observed effect on the antitumor immune response.

Cytokine secretion by inoculated tumor cells may augment the generation of an immune response by mechanisms fundamentally different from the exogenous systemic administration of the same cytokine. It also provides the theoretic advantage of continuous exposure to the cytokine at the tumor site, which is difficult to mimic even by repeated local cytokine injections or implantation of sustained release cytokine capsules. The majority of reports of cytokine gene transfection have involved the generation of immune animals by vaccination with genetically modified tumor cells (Tables 6.2–6.4). A few reports are emerging of successful treatment strategies of relatively small tumor burdens with genetically modified tumor cells (Table 6.5).

Table 6.2. *Immunologic characteristics of IL-1 and IL-2 transduced tumors*

Cytokine	Cell line	Amount secreted	Tumorigenic	Challenge immunity
IL-1α	Transformed fibroblasts	None	No	N.D.
IL-2	CT-26	40 U/ml	0/35 at 10^5 cells	Yes, at 2 weeks
			0/55 at 10^6 cells	25% at 4 weeks
			4/15 at 10^7 cells	
IL-2	CT-26	49–139 U/ml	21/46	45/82
IL-2	CT-26 plus IL-2-transduced fibroblasts		No	30/37
IL-2	CMS-5	30 U/ml	No, up to 2×10^6 cells	Yes, at 5 weeks
IL-2	4TO7	6 U/ml	1/6 at 2×10^5 cells	Yes
IL-2	J558L	40 U/ml	2/10 at 4×10^6 cells	2/5 at 2 weeks
				3/5 at 4 weeks
IL-2	B-16/F10	5000 U/ml	No	No
IL-2	HSNLV	5000 U/10^6 cells	6/12	N.D.
IL-2	MBT-2	10 U/ml	No	Yes, at 3.2×10^5 cells
IL-2	RLBA	10000 U/10^6 cells	N.D.	N.D.

Table 6.3. *Immunologic characteristics of IL-4, IL-5, IL-6 and IL-7 transduced tumor cells*

Cytokine	Tumor cell line	Amount secreted	Tumorigenic	Challenge immunity
IL-4	J558L	49 000 U/10^6 cells	No, 2 × 10^6 cells	No
IL-4	K485	5 600 U/10^6 cells	Yes	No
IL-4	J558L	75 U/ml	3/10	4/10 at 4 weeks
				2/10 at 2 weeks
IL-4	RENCA	1500 U/10^5 cells	0/10; 10^6 cells; yes, 10^5 cells	
IL-4	CT-26	1500 U/10^5 cells	0/10; 10^6 cells; yes, 10^5 cells	
IL-4	B-16	10 000 U/10^6 cells	No	No, 10^6 cells
IL-5	J558L	10–500 U/ml	Yes	N.D.
IL-5	TSA	20–500 U/ml	Yes	N.D.
IL-6	3LL	3 U/ml	Yes	6/7 at 10^5 cells
IL-6	B16-F10	400 ng/ml	Yes	No
IL-6	J558L	500 U/ml	Yes	N.D.
IL-6	205	25 U/10^5 cells 31/50	Yes	
IL-6	207	25 U/10^5 cells 0/27	Yes	
IL-7	203-glioma	52 U/ml	0/10 at 10^5 cells	Yes, in mice at 10^5 cells
			9/10 at 10^6 cells	
IL-7	FSA	20 ng/ml	No at 10^5 cells	N.D.
			Yes at 10^7 cells	
IL-7	J558L	50 U/ml	0/5 at 4 × 10^6 cells	2/10 at 2 weeks
				6/10 at 4 weeks
IL-7	TSA	50 U/ml	0/5 at 10^5 cells	N.D.

Table 6.4. *Immunologic characteristics of IFN-γ, TNF-α, G-CSF, and GM-CSF transduced tumor cells*

Cytokine	Tumor cell line	Amount secreted	Tumorigenic	Challenge immunity
IFN-γ	SP-1	256 U/ml	1/15 at 10^6 cells	No
IFN-γ	CT-26	8 U/ml	9/15 at 10^5 cells	N.D.
IFN-γ	C1300	50 U/ml	<5% at 3×10^6 cells	Yes
IFN-γ	D122	256 U/ml	No at 2×10^5 cells	Yes
IFN-γ	CMS-5	25 U/ml	0/3 at 5×10^5 cells 3/3 at 8×10^5 cells	Yes, i.v. Yes, 5/6 at 2 weeks
IFN-γ	J558L	125 ng/ml	0/10	3/10 at 2 weeks 0/10 at 4 weeks
IFN-γ	B16-F10	20 ng/ml	No	No
IFN-γ	MBT-2	150 ng/ml	No	Yes, at 4×10^5 cells
TNF-α	205	10 ng/24 hours	13/41 at 10^7 cells	Yes
TNF-α	J558L	40 pg/ml	12/30 at 5×10^6 cells	5/10 at 2 weeks 2/10 at 4 weeks
TNF-α	B16-F10	400 ng/ml	Yes	1/5
G-CSF	CT-26	1 ng/ml	0/10 at 10^7 cells	N.D.
GM-CSF	B16-F10	300 ng/ml	Yes	Yes
GM-CSF	CT-26	N.D.	N.D.	2/5
GM-CSF	CMS-5	N.D.	N.D.	5/5
GM-CSF	RENCA	N.D.	N.D.	3/5

IFN-γ, interferon-γ; TNF-α, tumor necrosis factor-α; G-CSF, granulocyte colony stimulation factor; GM-CSF, granulocyte macrophage colony stimulation factor.

Table 6.5. *Successful treatment of established tumor with genetically modified tumor cells*

Tumor type, dose	Time before vaccination (days)	Cytokine, amount secreted	Vaccination protocol	Survival advantage	Irradiated controls	Notes
MBT-2, 2 × 10^4 cells	7	IL-2, 10 U/ml	5 × 10^6 cells i.p. weekly ×4	Yes	Yes	60% long-term survivors
RENCA, 10^4 cells	6	IL-4 1500, U/10^5 cells	10^6 cells s.c. ×1	Yes	No	70% long-term survivors
RENCA, 10^4 cells	9	IL-4 1500, U/10^5 cells	10^6 cells s.c. ×1	Yes	No	20% long-term survivors
D122, 2 × 10^5 cells	11	IL-6, 3 U/ml	2 × 10^6 cells i.p. weekly ×6	N.D.	Yes	Vaccination not effective in nude mice
D122, 2 × 10^5 cells	11	IFN-γ, 256 U/ml	2 × 10^6 cells i.p. weekly ×5	N.D.	Yes	
BL6-F10, 5 × 10^4 cells	3	GM-CSF, 200 ng/ml	4 × 10^6 cells ×1	Yes	Yes	80% long-term survivors
BL6-F10, 1 × 10^5 cells	3	GM-CSF, 300 ng/ml	4 × 10^6 cells ×1	Yes	Yes	40% long-term survivors
BERH-2, 2 × 10^7 cells	10	(Fused with B cells)	5 × 10^6 cells ×1	Yes	Yes	100% long-term survivors

Interleukin 2

Interleukin 2 is one of the more critical cytokines in cellular immune responses and is secreted by CD4 T cells in response to antigen binding. Antigen is presented to CD4 cells by antigen-presenting cells expressing other costimulatory ligands which facilitate cellular interactions (i.e., CD2/LFA-3, LFA-1/ICAM-1, or CD28/B7 binding). The effects of IL-2 are mediated by a heterotrimeric high-affinity receptor (IL-2R). The receptor is usually only expressed after induction on T cells, B cells, and monocytes. IL-2 can induce production of IL-1, IL-6, tumor necrosis factor (TNF), and interferon by other immune cells. In addition, exposure to IL-2 can increase the cytotoxicity of T cells and natural killer (NK) cells. Systemic administration of IL-2 can stimulate a variety of therapeutic immune responses in vivo to infectious agents such as malaria, herpes virus, and rabies, and can mediate the regression of established tumors (Mulé et al., 1987; Rosenberg et al., 1985; Kroemer et al., 1991; Swain, 1991). Thus the elaboration of IL-2 by tumor cells may stimulate both T cell proliferation and activation at the tumor site. In addition, IL-2 secretion by tumor cells may overcome the need for a CD4 T cell response to generate antitumor immunity.

The genetic modification of tumor cells to secrete IL-2 has been extensively studied (see Table 6.2). Fearon et al. reported on the immunobiology of two murine tumors genetically modified to secrete IL-2 (Fearon et al., 1990). The CT-26 tumor was modified to secrete 40 U/ml of IL-2. The IL-2-secreting cells demonstrated reduced tumorigenicity at a dose of 10^7 cells. Rejection of the transfected tumor cells was demonstrated to be primarily dependent on CD4 T cells. Protective immunity was afforded to 100% of the mice at two weeks after vaccination with 10^6 IL-2-secreting CT26 cells. However, four weeks postvaccination, immunity was only noted in 30% of the mice. Similar experiments performed with the poorly immunogenic BL6 melanoma genetically modified to secrete IL-2 in essentially the same amount demonstrated no tumor growth at doses up to 10^6 cells, and five of nine animals were protected at two weeks from a subsequent challenge of parental cells. These studies demonstrated that IL-2 secretion by a tumor could provide short-term protective immunity.

Gansbacher et al. reported their results with the CMS-5 tumor modified to secrete 30 U/ml of IL-2 (Gansbacher et al., 1990a). They observed no tumor growth of the IL-2-secreting cells at doses up to 10^6 cells. Tumor-free mice were immune to rechallenge with 3×10^5 parental tumor cells six weeks later. The IL-2-secreting cells were able to mediate the rejection of up to 8×10^5 unmodified cells when implanted at the same site.

Dranoff et al. reported on studies with the B16 melanoma engineered to secrete high levels of IL-2 (5000 U/ml) (Dranoff et al., 1993). They found that while this high level of IL-2 secretion abrogated tumorigenicity, no protective immunity was generated. It was speculated that 'nonspecific' killing of the tumor was caused by this high level of IL-2 secretion without the induction of tumor-reactive T cells.

Two separate reports studied the mechanisms of abrogated tumorigenicity of the J558L plasmacytoma which was engineered to secrete 40 U/ml of IL-2 (Hock et al., 1993a, 1993b). In the first report, IL-2-secreting cells were able to protect 40% of mice from a dose of 2×10^6 cells at two weeks and 60% of mice at four weeks (Hock et al., 1993b). However, the protective effect of IL-2-secreting cells was not as large as that of the parental J558L cells administered with the adjuvant *Corynebacterium parvum*. Hock et al. also explored the mechanism of rejection of the IL-2-secreting cells (Hock et al., 1993b). Nude mice (T cell deficient), SCID mice (T and B cell deficient), SCID/beige mice (T cell, B cell, and NK cell deficient), and NIH III mice (T cell deficient, NK cell deficient and X-linked immunodeficient) were not able to reject IL-2-secreting cells, in contrast to immunocompetent mice. However, the tumors that eventually grew in these immunocompromised mice grew with delayed kinetics and had greatly decreased levels of cytokine production. Depletion in normal mice of NK activity by administering asialo-GM-1 antibodies only partially restored the tumor growth kinetics of IL-2-secreting cells. Depletion of CD4 T cells did not restore the tumorigenicity of IL-2-secreting cells, but depletion of CD8 cells did. Histologic analysis of the regressing tumors revealed a predominant CD8 T cell infiltrate. These studies demonstrated that CD8 T cells appear to be the primary mediators of tumor rejection. Additional unidentified cells may play an important role in immediate rejection as well.

Vaccination with IL-2-secreting cells has been able to treat disseminated malignancy in one report (see Table 6.5; Connor et al., 1993). A transfected MBT-2 cell line secreting between 9 and 20 units of IL-2 was isolated, and shown to be nontumorigenic in doses up to 10^5 cells. Vaccination with IL-2-secreting cells was able to generate animals immune to a challenge of up to 3.2×10^5 cells three weeks after vaccination. Treatment of established seven-day tumor with four doses of irradiated 5×10^6 IL-2-secreting cells was able to cure 60% of animals. By contrast, treatment with irradiated parental cells was not able to eradicate tumor. The animals that were cured of their tumor were able to reject a subsequent challenge of the parental MBT-2 cells. This study demonstrated that treatment with IL-2-secreting cells prolonged survival of mice bearing disseminated tumors. No data were provided on how therapy with genetically modified cells would compare to unmodified cells with adjuvant. However, this is one of the few studies that provide a rationale for its application in clinical therapy.

A recent report examined the ability of IL-2-secreting fibroblasts to serve as adjuvants for CT26 immunization (Shawler et al., 1995). CT26 cells were genetically modified to secrete between 49 and 166 U/ml of IL-2. The IL-2-secreting cells were less tumorigenic than parental tumor, although 21/46 (46%) of the animals inoculated with IL-2-secreting CT26 cells developed tumors. When parental CT26 cells were admixed with IL-2-secreting fibroblasts, none of the animals developed tumors at the vaccination site. The IL-2-secreting fibroblasts provided levels of protective immunity similar to those of the IL-2-secreting CT26 cells. As fibroblasts are considerably easier to grow and transduce with viral vectors than most primary tumor cell lines, the genetic modification of fibroblasts may prove more clinically feasible than the modification of primary tumor cells.

Interleukin 4

The major source of IL-4 in vivo is CD4 T lymphocytes. While originally identified as a B cell growth factor, subsequent studies have demonstrated that it can also stimulate the proliferation of T cells. IL-4 receptors are expressed on a wide variety of cell types. Knock-out mice deficient in IL-4 secretion demonstrate a virtual absence of IgG1-mediated and IgE-mediated immune responses. In-vitro assays have demonstrated the ability of IL-4 to induce Class I expression. Significantly, IL-4 has been reported to increase the expansion of immunologically specific tumor infiltrating lymphocytes (TIL) from human melanomas (Kawakami, Rosenberg and Lotze, 1988).

Secretion of IL-4 by tumor cells to enhance host antitumor immunity has been studied by two groups of investigators (see Table 6.3; Tepper, Pattengale and Leder, 1989; Golumbek et al., 1991; Tepper, Coffman and Leder, 1992). Tepper et al. noted that IL-4 overexpression in transgeneic animals caused an allergic-like autoimmune disease (Tepper et al., 1990). The same investigators engineered tumor cells to secrete IL-4 (Tepper et al., 1989). Using a genomic clone of IL-4, they generated a J558L cell line that secreted approximately 50 000 U/ml IL-4 and a breast carcinoma cell line that secreted 4000 U/ml IL-4. The higher secreting cell line did not grow in immune-competent animals, nor in nude animals, suggesting that abrogation of tumorigencity was not a T-cell-mediated phenomenon. Histologic analysis of the tumors during the rejection phase demonstrated an eosinophilic infiltrate, and a subsequent study showed that depletion of the animals of eosinophils and mature granulocytes restored tumorigenicity (Tepper et al., 1992). This report also demonstrated that animals rejecting their tumor were not immune to a subsequent challenge with parental tumor. Modification of the poorly immunogenic B16-F10 to secrete IL-4 also abrogated tumorigenicity of this cell line, but animals that rejected the IL-4-secreting tumor were not immune to a challenge of parental tumor. The plasmacytoma cell line was demonstrated. to be rejected by three types of immune-deficient mice (nude, Bg/nude/xid, and SCID), providing further evidence that these high IL-4-secreting cell lines are rejected in a non-T-cell-dependent manner.

Golumbek et al. reported their ability to treat established disease with a different tumor modified to secrete IL-4 (Golumbek et al., 1991). They transfected the RENCA renal cell tumor with an IL-4 construct and obtained a tumor clone which secreted 1500 U/24 hours of IL-4. The tumor cell line secreting IL-4 had abrogated tumorigenicity in immune-competent mice. In contrast to the report by the other group, these tumors grew in SCID and nude mice; however, the time until tumor outgrowth was 80–100 days in immunocompromised animals, and the outgrowing tumors were not analyzed for IL-4 secretion. Histologic analysis of the regressing tumors at five days revealed the characteristic eosinophilic infiltrate similar to that observed by others; but at ten days a T cell infiltrate was observed. The animals inoculated with RENCA–IL-4 cells were immune to a challenge of 10^5 wild-type cells, suggesting that IL-4 gene modification had provided a degree of protective immunity. Depletion of CD8 cells during the immunization with modified cells abrogated the ability to resist a subsequent tumor challenge; while depletion of CD4 cells during the immunization only partially abrogated effectiveness of the immunization. When 10^4 parental cells were inoculated subcutaneously, vaccination with IL-4 transfected tumor cells six and nine days after tumor inoculation was able to cure 70% and 20% of the animals, respectively. This latter study did not compare therapy with IL-4-secreting cells to vaccination with parental cells or parental cells admixed with an adjuvant.

IL-4 has been reported to augment the immunogenicity of the poorly immunogenic BL6 melanoma by Krauss et al. (1994). In these studies, a recombinant retrovirus vector was used to modify a subclone of the B16 melanoma. Two IL-4-secreting cells lines were isolated, one secreting 39 U/ml of IL-4, and one secreting 80 U/ml of IL-4. Both IL-4-secreting cell lines grew more slowly than parental cells in mice, but retained tumorigenicity in all animals tested. Lymph nodes draining a progressively growing tumor contain sensitized T lymphocytes that, when cultured ex vivo with anti-CD3 monoclonal antibody and expanded in IL-2, can mediate the regression of macroscopic tumor burdens. Both IL-4-secreting cell lines enhanced the induction of tumor-reactive T cells in the draining lymph node, as compared to vector-only modified cells or unmodified parental cells. These T cells significantly reduced tumor burden.

For both IL-2 and IL-4 gene transfection, enough studies with various tumor cell lines have been reported to draw some conclusions. In many ways, cytokine gene transfection of tumor appears to modulate host immunity in a fashion similar to the use of classical bacterial immune adjuvants such as *C. parvum*. At high levels of secretion, nonspecific tumor cell destruction occurs without the generation of systemic immunity to the tumor. At low levels of cytokine secretion, it appears to increase the immunogenicity of the tumor. At the very lowest levels of secretion of cytokine, the induction of immunity appears less complete. Thus, unlike conventional pharmacology where 'more is better' in terms of an antitumor response, careful dose titration may be required to address adequately the most potent combination of cytokines to generate immunity.

Interleukin 6

The biologic activity ascribed to IL-6 was originally isolated as interferon β-2 from fibroblasts. Subsequent studies have demonstrated that IL-6 can stimulate the proliferation of T cells activated with lectins, and can induce cytolytic T cell differentiation. Adminstration of human IL-6 to mice has been reported to mediate the reduction of pulmonary and hepatic micrometastases, and this effect has been demonstrated to be mediated by T cells. IL-6 also has a variety of effects on the proliferation of hematopoietic stem cells. In addition, IL-6 has been implicated in the pathogenesis of multiple myeloma. In a susceptible strain of mice, constitutive IL-6 production can result in clonally derived malignant myelomas. Thus transfection of IL-6 in tumors of hematopoietic origin could potentially augment their growth. However, the local secretion if IL-6 by other types of tumor cells has the potential for mediating T cell proliferation and differentiation at the tumor site.

IL-6-transfected tumor cells have also been demonstrated to be capable of treating established disease, as reported by Porgador et al. (1992). Using a clone of the Lewis lung carcinoma (D122), they established a cell line which secreted 3 U/ml of IL-6 (see Tables 6.3 and 6.5). They demonstrated that this cell line generated fewer spontaneous metastases when injected in the footpad, and grew less well in the lung when injected intravenously. Neither immune-competent nor nude mice rejected the IL-6-secreting cells. IL-6-secreting cells when irradiated were able to provide some protective immunity over immunization with parental cells. In addition, the burden of lung metastases was reduced when animals were inoculated with IL-6-secreting tumors three times, starting on day 11 after establishment of tumor. While survival of the mice was not reported, this study suggested some therapeutic effect of immunization with IL-6-secreting cells as compared to immunization with parental cells.

Mullen et al. recently reported their results with IL-6 transfected tumors (Mullen et al., 1992). They modified two weakly immunogenic sarcomas, MCA 205 and MCA 207, to secrete between 20 and 25 U IL-6/24 hours. IL-6-secreting MCA 207 cells were rejected by normal but not by nude mice, while MCA 205–IL-6 cells were not rejected, but did exhibit slower in-vivo growth characteristics than the parental cells. MCA 205 cells secreting IL-6 were able to reduce slightly the mean number of five-day-old pulmonary metastases, although the magnitude of this effect did not reach statistical significance. Specificity of immunity was demonstrated by showing that mice immunized with MCA 207–IL-6 tumors efficiently rejected MCA 207 but not MCA 205 tumors; while hosts immunized with MCA 205–IL-6 tumors efficiently rejected MCA 205 but not MCA 207 tumors. Further studies may elucidate the role that IL-6 gene transfection can play in generating antitumor immunity.

Interleukin 7

Interleukin 7 was first identified as a factor capable of supporting the growth of pre-B cells in the absence of supporting bone marrow stromal cells. Subsequent cloning of the murine and human cDNAs, as well as the receptors, has provided more information regarding the IL-7/IL-7R system. To date, bone marrow stromal cells, fetal thymus, and cultured thymic stroma have been demonstrated to be sources of IL-7 protein, while IL-7 RNA has been detected in those tissues as well as spleen, adult thymus, kidney, and fetal liver. Both T and B cells respond to IL-7 by proliferation. In addition, IL-7 has been demonstrated to generate LAK and NK activity, as well as to induce tumoricidal activity of macrophages. Thus IL-7 elaboration by tumors has several potential mechanisms of action.

Secretion of IL-7 by tumors has been reported by three separate groups to increase immunogenicity (Hock et al., 1991; Aoki et al., 1992; McBride et al., 1992). Hock et al. reported on the transfection with IL-7 of the plasmacytoma cells J558L, to generate cell lines which produced between 4 and 50 U/ml of IL-7 (Hock et al., 1991). The 50 U/ml secreting cell lines were efficiently rejected after subcutaneous inoculation by immune-competent, but not nude, mice, at doses up to 4×10^6 cells. Using antibody depletion of immune cell subsets, they demonstrated that CD8 T cells, CD4 T cells, and complement receptor type 3 positive cells (predominantly monocytes, macrophages, and neutrophils) were necessary for tumor rejection, as depletion of any of these subsets restored tumor growth. A subsequent report by this same group demonstrated that between 40% and 80% of the mice could reject the parental tumor at four weeks after vaccination with genetically modified cells (Hock et al., 1993b).

Aoki et al. reported on the modification of the glioblastoma cell line 203 to secrete IL-7 (Aoki et al., 1992). They reported complete rejection of a clone that secreted IL-7 (50 U/ml) up to a tumor cell dose of 2.5×10^5 cells; at doses of 10^6–10^7 cells, all of the animals developed tumors. Mice that rejected the genetically modified tumor were immune to a subsequent challenge of parental tumor. A comparison of these results to those obtained with irradiated cells alone was not made. In additional studies, tumorigenicity was restored by CD8 T cell depletion, but not by CD4 and NK cell depletion.

McBride et al. also reported their findings with the FSA sarcoma modified to secrete approximately 20 ng IL-7/ml (McBride et al., 1992). IL-7 secretion by the tumor cells increased the number of cells required for 100% tumorigenicity from 10^4 to 10^7 cells. Nude mice had similar tumorigenic doses of parental and IL-7-secreting cells. No studies to evaluate the development of systemic immunity in animals inoculated with IL-7-secreting tumors were performed. Of note, they demonstrated that exogenous IL-7 could slow tumor growth.

Interleukin 12

Recently, Tahara and colleagues described the effects of IL-12 secretion on tumorigenicity and immunogenicity (Tahara et al., 1995). A novel viral vector, TFG, was constructed, which utilizes a viral ribosomal re-entry site to allow for the translation of a tricistronic RNA in mammalian cells. Bulk selected cells transduced with this vector secreted between 9 ng/ml and 100 ng/ml of IL-12. Interleukin 12 secretion by MCA 205 or MCA 207 tumor cells abrogated tumorigenicity. In therapy experiments with MCA 207–IL-12-secreting cells, therapy at day 0 eliminated tumor at a distant site in 80% of the animals, while therapy at day 12 eliminated tumors only in 20% of the animals. Depletion of all T cells (CD4 and CD8) and NK cells with monoclonal antibodies completely restored tumorigenicity of the IL-12-secreting cells, but depletion of any one of these immune cell subsets was only marginally effective. Blockade of interferon-γ (IFN-γ) but not of tumor necrosis factor-α (TNF-α), partially restored tumorigenicity. Thus IL-12 secretion by tumor cells demonstrated substantial antitumor activity.

Interferon-γ

Interferon-γ was first recognized for its antiviral activity in 1965. The subsequent cloning of the human and murine interferon genes and interferon receptor genes has added substantially to knowledge of the role of this mediator in the immune response. IFN-γ is produced by CD8 and some CD4 T cells. It is biologically active only as a homodimer. The IFN-γ receptor is ubiquitously expressed. IFN-γ has been demonstrated to enhance MHC Class I expression and induce MHC Class II expression. Local production of IFN-γ tends to favor the development of cell-mediated rather than humoral immunity. Both the upregulation of MHC expression and the augmentation of a cell-mediated immune response suggest that secretion of IFN-γ by tumor cells will favorably modulate the antitumor immune response.

Several investigators have published reports regarding the ability of IFN-γ to modulate the immunogenicity of tumors (see Table 6.4; Watanabe et al., 1989; Gansbacher et al., 1990b; Esumi et al., 1991; Restifo et al., 1992; Dranoff et al., 1993; Hock et al., 1993b; Porgador et al., 1993). Watanabe et al. reported that the genetic modification of C1300 cells to secrete IFN-γ decreased tumorigenicity at a dose of 10^6 cells (Watanabe et al., 1989). Mice that rejected tumors were immune to a challenge with parental tumor. Depletion of immune cell subsets with monoclonal antibodies revealed that mice depleted of CD8 cells lost the ability to reject gene-modified tumor cells, while those with depletion of macrophages or NK cells retained the lack of tumor growth by IFN-γ-secreting cells.

Gansbacher et al. reported abrogation of CMS-5 tumorigenicity by IFN-γ gene-modified cells at doses up to 8×10^5 cells (Gansbacher et al., 1990b). The majority of mice challenged with 2×10^5 parental tumor cells subsequently rejected the tumor. IFN-γ-transduced cells demonstrated upregulated MHC Class I expression. In another study, Esumi et al. transfected SP1 cells such that they produced up to 256 U/ml of IFN-γ (Esumi et al. 1991). The secreting cells demonstrated abrogation of tumorigenicity at doses up to 10^6 cells. However, none of the animals exhibited resistance to a subsequent challenge of parental tumor cells at a dose as low as 10^4 cells. A second tumor, CT26, modified to secrete IFN-γ, retained tumorigenicity.

Restifo et al. reported on the immunobiologic effects of IFN-γ transfection of the poorly immunogenic MCA 101 fibrosarcoma (Restifo et al., 1992). Although IFN-γ-transduced tumor cells did not secrete detectable IFN-γ and grew progressively, they were able to isolate antitumor reactive tumor-infiltrating lymphocytes (TIL) from the genetically modified tumors established in vivo, which was not possible with the parental tumor. The TIL derived from the IFN-γ-modified tumors mediated regression of parental pulmonary metastases in an adoptive immunotherapy model. These investigators also presented data demonstrating that IFN-γ-transfected MCA 101 tumor cells expressed increased MHC Class I molecules and were able to present viral antigens to CD8 CTL, which the parental tumor line failed to do. This suggested that IFN-γ-transfected tumor cells may be rendered more immunogenic, namely by presenting increased amounts of tumor antigen.

Treatment of established tumor by IFN-γ-secreting lung cancer D122 was reported by Porgador et al. (1993). IFN-γ-secreting transfectants exhibited delayed growth in both immunocompetent and nude mice. Interestingly, IFN-γ-nonsecreting tumors were slightly better than IFN-γ-secreting tumors at immunizing naive animals. However, when used for active specific immunotherapy of established metastases, IFN-γ-secreting clones were slightly more active than nonsecreting clones. This suggested that IFN-γ-transduced cells can serve to eliminate small amounts of tumor, although this was evident only in this one animal model. The fact that IFN-γ-secreting clones grew significantly slower in nude mice indicated that mechanisms other than classic T-cell-mediated immunity may be operative.

Tumor necrosis factor-α

Tumor necrosis factor-α is produced by macrophages and numerous other cell types after a wide range of physiologic and pathologic stimuli. Almost all cells express one or both of the TNF receptors. TNF and IL-1 appear to have an overlapping spectrum of activity in vivo, including activation and differentiation of macrophages. Secretion of TNF by tumors may therefore augment the local macrophage cytocidal or cytostatic activity. TNF secretion may also stimulate the infiltration of T cells, as well as the influx of nonspecific inflammatory cells such as NK cells and polymorphonuclear leucocytes in vivo.

TNF-α-transfected into tumor was reported to cause a quicker death of nude mice inoculated with the genetically modified tumors, potentially implicating release of TNF-α as a mediator of tumor cachexia (Oliff et al., 1987). Other investigators have reported an alteration in tumorigenicity by TNF-α transfection in different tumor models (see Table 6.4; Blankenstein et al., 1991; Asher et al., 1991; Teng et al., 1991). Blankenstein et al. reported on the modification of J558L to secrete 50 pg/ml of TNF-α. In this report, 60% of animals were able to reject 5×10^6 TNF-α-secreting cells. J558L tumors secreting TNF-α grew in nude, SCID, SCID/beige, and nude/Xid/beige mice. Animals depleted of CD8 T cells but not of CD4 cells efficiently rejected

TNF-α-secreting tumors. Asher et al. reported on the weakly immunogenic tumor MCA 205 engineered to secrete between 500 and 10 000 pg/24 hours of TNF-α (Asher et al., 1991). Clones secreting higher amounts of TNF-α grew and regressed in the majority of cases, resulting in animals immune to subsequent challenges with parental tumor. Depletion of either CD4 or CD8 T cells restored tumorigenicity. Teng et al. reported that transfection of a skin tumor, PRO 4L.7, with a TNF-α expression construct inhibited tumor growth in nude mice (Teng et al., 1991). This suggested that some non-T cell mechanisms were responsible for growth inhibition by TNF-α-transfected tumors. No conclusions could be drawn concerning immunity to subsequent tumor challenge since suitable experiments were not performed. In another study, Dranoff et al. reported that the poorly immunogenic BL6-F10 melanoma transfected with the TNF-α gene (secreting 400 ng/ml of TNF-α) grew progressively in immunocompetent mice (Dranoff et al., 1993). These latter observations indicate that, despite relatively high levels of TNF-α secretion, the growth of certain tumors (i.e., possibly poorly immunogenic tumors) is not affected.

Granulocyte colony stimulating factor

Granulocyte colony stimulating factor (G-CSF) genetic modification has been reported to increase immunogenicity by Colombo et al. (see Table 6.4; Colombo et al. 1991). They reported that CT-26 cells modified to secrete 900 pg/ml of G-CSF demonstrated abrogated tumorigenicity at doses up to 10^7 cells. Mixtures of G-CSF-secreting cells and unmodified parental cells failed to grow in normal mice, nude mice, and NK-cell-depleted mice; but grew in sublethally irradiated mice. Further studies by these same investigators revealed that depletion of CD8 cells or depletion of mature neutrophils restored tumorigenicity (Stoppacciaro et al., 1993). Blockade of IFN-γ by monoclonal antibody adminstration also restored tumorigenicity. Whether or not the animals developed systemic immunity was not reported; nor was a treatment strategy using gene-modified cells presented.

Granulocyte macrophage colony stimulating factor

Granulocyte macrophage colony stimulating factor (GM-CSF) cytokine gene transfection has been reported to stimulate potent immunity to tumor when transduced into the poorly immunogenic BL6-F10 melanoma (Dranoff et al., 1993). Using a retroviral vector that is highly efficient at secreting protein, these investigators compared the immunogenicity of BL6-F10 transfected with several different immunoregulatory proteins which included IL-2, IL-4, IL-5, IL-6, GM-CSF, IFN-γ, IL-1 receptor antagonist, ICAM-1, CD2 and TNF-α. Bulk retrovirus transduced cells were studied, and in some cases, vector was present in only 10% of cells used in the vaccine. Only IL-2-secreting cells were nontumorigenic, but in contrast to studies reported by others, the mice that rejected IL-2-secreting cells were not immune to a challenge with parental cells. Combinations of IL-2 and all of the other cytokines were tested, and only IL-2 in addition to GM-CSF yielded a significant proportion (60%) of animals immune to challenge with parental tumor. Using irradiated, singly transduced tumor cell vaccines, only GM-CSF generated a significant proportion of mice immune to parental tumor. Treatment with a single dose of irradiated GM-CSF-producing cells was able to produce long-term survival of 40% of mice with subcutaneous tumor established three days earlier by the inoculation of 10^5 parental cells. Cellular depletion analysis of immune mice revealed that depletion of either CD4 or CD8 cells restored tumorigencity, while depletion of NK cells only restored tumorigencity in 30% of mice. It was demonstrated that inoculation of irradiated CT-26, CMS-5, RENCA, and WP-4 (a clone of MCA 205) tumor cells could result in immune animals, indicating their weakly immunogenic characteristics. However, by varying the vaccine and challenge dose of cells, Dranoff et al. could demonstrate enhanced immunogenicity of GM-CSF-secreting CT-26, RENCA, and CMS-5 cells. This exhaustive series of experiments illustrates some of the problems inherent in screening cytokines for enhancement of improved efficacy of tumor cell vaccines.

Arca and colleagues reported the effects of GM-CSF-secreting tumor on the sensitization of regional lymph nodes for use in adoptive immunotherapy (Arca et al., 1996). A weakly immunogenic subclone of the B16 melanoma was modified to secrete GM-CSF. The GM-CSF-secreting tumor cells grew only slightly slower than the parental, unmodified cells, and killed all of the animals within three weeks of inoculation. Unlike the previous study, vaccination with irradiated GM-CSF-secreting tumor cells failed to protect against challenge with wild-type tumor, demonstrating the weak immunogenicity of this B16 subline. T lymphocytes cultured from the lymph node draining the GM-CSF-secreting tumor demonstrated enhanced therapeutic reactivity against established pulmonary metastases of parental tumor. The percentage of macrophages and neutrophils was greatly increased in the draining lymph node, suggesting that GM-CSF secretion by the tumor may lead to enhanced antigen presentation by these cells. GM-CSF-secreting tumor cells were more potent than the admixture of *C. parvum* and tumor at sensitizing T cells in the regional lymph node. Furthermore, comparison to IL-4-

secreting tumor cells revealed that the GM-CSF-secreting tumor cells were more active at sensitizing T cells in the regional lymph node. Thus, GM-CSF secretion by tumor cells has been the most promising adjuvant identified to date for sensitizing T cells for adoptive immunotherapy. These murine experiments have led to a proposed Phase I human clinical trial at the University of Michigan, in which autologous melanoma cells will be transduced to secrete GM-CSF, and subsequently used to prime regional lymph nodes. The lymph nodes containing tumor-sensitized T cells will be retrieved for anti-CD3/IL-2 activation, and then the T cells will be adoptively transferred back to the patient for therapy.

Tumor transfection with other immunoregulatory genes

Costimulatory B7 ligand

The presentation of neoantigens outside of the thymus can induce either tolerance or immunity. The absence of costimulation at the time of antigen presentation will result in an anergic T cell and peripheral tolerance; while the presence of a second signal will generate a functionally active T cell and immunity. Recent insights in T cell biology have demonstrated that one possible second signal for IL-2 production by CD4 T cells is the engagement of CD28 expressed on T cells with B7 present on antigen-presenting cells (Schwartz, 1992). Therefore, in MHC Class II positive tumors, expression of B7 by the tumor cell may stimulate IL-2 production by CD4 T cells and lead to immunity directed at peptides displayed by the tumor cell. Injection of a soluble B7 competitor (CTLA4-Ig) inhibits the immune response to both soluble antigens and particulate antigens. Treatment with CTLA4-Ig can delay and/or prevent the rejection of allografts, further stressing the importance of this counter-receptor for costimulation.

Transfection of the costimulatory B7 gene into tumors has been reported by two groups, with divergent results using the same tumor model (Chen et al., 1992; Townsend and Allison, 1993). Townsend and Allison generated B7-expressing transfectants of the K1735 melanoma, and demonstrated that the transfectants were able to provide in-vitro costimulation, while the parental tumor and control transfectants could not (Townsend and Allison, 1993). The B7 transfectants generally grew and regressed in vivo, while the control transfectants grew progressively. Approximately 90% of the mice that had been exposed to the B7 transfectant were immune to a subsequent challenge with the parental tumor 25 days later. T cell subset depletion analyses revealed that rejection of B7 transfection tumors was primarily dependent on CD8 T cells, although depletion of CD4 cells caused tumor growth in a proportion of the animals. Comparative experiments of generating immune animals with nontransfected tumor cells were not reported to assess the native immunogenicity of this tumor. Furthermore, experiments utilizing the B7 transfectants in the treatment of established disease were not performed.

Chen et al. reported their findings with transfecting the B7 gene utilizing the same melanoma, K1735 (Chen et al., 1992). Despite efficient expression of B7 on the cell surface, the transfectants grew progressively in mice. However, transfection of the E7 human papilloma virus antigen in addition to B7 resulted in tumors that grew and regressed. This suggested that besides B7, a strong tumor-associated antigen was required to initiate a host immune response. The regression could be blocked by depleting the mice of CD4 T cells, but not of CD8 T cells. In-vivo blockade of B7 with CTLA4-Ig also blocked tumor rejection. Animals treated with E7/B7-positive tumor cells were immune to challenges of E7-positive tumors, but not of the parental tumor. Finally, E7/B7 tumors were able to cure approximately 70% of mice inoculated with established E7-positive metastatic tumors. This effect was not evident against the parental tumor.

Chen and colleagues reported in 1994 that inherent tumor immunogenicity was the major determining factor as to the strength of the effect of B7 gene transfection on enhancing immunogenicity (Chen et al., 1994). They constructed a retrovirus vector encoding for murine B7 and used it to transduce several tumor cell lines of differing immunogenicities. Tumors were defined as either possessing transplantation immunogenicity, or lacking such immunogenicity by standard vaccination/challenge experiments. Minimal initiating tumor dose alone is not an adequate measure of tumor immunogenicity; a dramatic (1–2 log) increase in minimal tumor-initiating dose after vaccination is also required to define a tumor as immunogenic. EL-4 and P815 tumors both required multiple boosts with irradiated cells to be defined as immunogenic, but similar boosts with the other tumors (MCA 101, MCA 102, Ag 104, and B16) did not increase tumor immunogenicity measurably. Chen et al. constructed a retrovirus vector encoding for murine B7 and used it to transduce several tumor cell lines of differing immunogenicities. Similar levels of B7 expression were obtained on the different tumor cell lines, as measured by flow cytometry. Tumorigenicity was abrogated by B7 expression in the more immunogenic RMA, EL-4, E6B2, and P815 tumor cell lines. Tumorigenicity was unchanged by B7 expression in the less immunogenic MCA 101, MCA 102, B16, and Ag 104 cell lines. Similarly, protective immunity could be induced with B7 transduced EL4 and P815 cells, but not with B7 transduced MCA 101, MCA 102, B16, or Ag 104 cells. Transduced

EL-4 cells could treat four-day established parental tumor. Thus tumors that possess inherent transplantation immunogenicity were augmented with B7 gene transfection, while those that lacked transplantation immunogenicity were not augmented with B7 transfection. This exhaustive series of experiments demonstrates the relatively modest effect of B7-1 transfection on enhancing tumor immunogenicity.

Heat shock protein

Lukacs et al., reported that transfection of the heat shock protein (hsp65) from *Mycobacterium leprae* increased tumor immunogenicity (Lukacs et al., 1993). J774 cells expressing hsp65 were nontumorigenic in immunocompetent mice at doses up to 10^7 cells and in nude mice at similar doses. Immunized immunocompetent mice could reject parental tumor, while immunized nude mice were not immune to parental tumor. Irradiated vector-only cells were able to induce immunity in 50% of the mice. Purified hsp65 admixed with tumor cells was not able to abrogate tumorigencity, indicating the protein needed to be present on the tumor cell. This first report of hsp enhancing immunogenicity represents a novel approach to generating an antitumor response. Since many hsps are protein chaperones, it is postulated that this protein may be functioning to increase immunogenicity by augmenting mutated oncogene presentation.

Fusion of B cells and tumor cells

In a recent study, the addition of a combination of immunoregulatory molecules to a tumor cell line was reported to decrease tumorigenicity and was effective in the treatment of established tumor. The addition of these immunoregulatory molecules was accomplished by the fusion of activated B cells with tumor cells utilizing polyethylene glycol (Guo et al., 1994). Activated rat B cells were fused to a rat hepatocellular carcinoma (BERH-2) and subsequently selected for expression of both tumor cell epitopes and B cell epitopes with polyclonal sera. As compared to the parental BERH-2 tumor cells, the fused cells demonstrated increased expression of MHC Class I, MHC Class II, costimulatory molecule B7, lymphocyte function antigen 1 (LFA-1), and ICAM-1. The fused BERH-2 cells failed to produce tumors in doses of up to 2×10^6 cells, and animals that had rejected these cells were immune to an intrahepatic challenge of 5×10^6 parental BERH-2 cells. Furthermore, rats injected ten days earlier with 2×10^7 cells were able to be cured of tumors when inoculated with 5×10^6 fused BERH-2 cells, but not when inoculated with parental cells. Rejection of the fused tumor cells was dependent on both CD4 and CD8 T cells, since depletion of either cellular subset restored tumorigencity of the fused BERH-2 cells. Elimination of tumor after immunization was only dependent on CD8 T cells. While it remains to be determined which B cell molecules are critical for the observed enhancement of immunogenicity, the dramatic results seen in this tumor model suggest that a combination of immunoregulatory genes and proteins may be more effective than a single class of molecules.

Conclusion

A plethora of animal studies have demonstrated that gene addition can increase the immunogenicity of tumors. Only a few trials have demonstrated therapeutic efficacy in the treatment of established disease with genetically modified tumor cell vaccines. To date, vaccination with gene-modified tumor cells has not been able to demonstrate enhanced host immunity over vaccination with tumor cells and conventional bacterial adjuvants. Given the large number of patients who have been unsuccessfully treated with tumor vaccines with or without bacterial adjuvants in the past, it seems unlikely at the current stage that any of the human trials with genetically modified tumor cells will produce significant therapeutic results. Nevertheless, the information derived from basic and clinical studies of genetically modified tumor cells as immunogens will enhance our knowledge regarding the mechanisms involved in host immunity to tumors. Ultimately, the use of genetically modified tumor vaccines may have its optimal therapeutic role as an adjuvant treatment for cancer patients who have had removal of all gross tumor and are at high risk for recurrent disease from micrometastases. Patients with unresectable advanced tumors may require additional therapeutic approaches in conjunction with genetically modified tumor vaccines. One such approach may be the use of cytokines to modulate the host systemic response to genetically engineered tumor vaccines. Another approach may be to employ genetically modified tumor vaccines to elicit immune cells which can be further expanded for adoptive immunotherapy.

Besides the treatment of established disease, prevention of spontaneous (or mutagen-induced) malignancies through vaccination also holds theoretical promise. Historically, vaccination has been most useful in preventing disease rather than in treating established disease. Elimination of sequelae of infectious diseases provides one route for the prevention of cancer. Vaccination against hepatitis B has the potential of eliminating chronic active hepatitis as a cause of hepatocellular carcinoma. Development of an effective vaccine against Epstein–Barr virus may decrease the incidence of malignancies such as nasopharyngeal carcinoma and Burkitt's lymphoma. Similarly, development of vaccines to prevent the major human retrovirus infections (i.e., HIV and HTLV) would eliminate those diseases as etiologic agents of malignancy. With increasing knowledge about the molecular events which occur during carcinogenesis, immunological approaches to specific molecular targets may potentially block the development of a malignancy. The identification of novel chimeric proteins such as bcr/abl in chronic myelogenous leukemia provides an identifiable target for the immune response. In addition, shared mutations in oncogenes such as *ras* provide a theoretic basis for preventing malignancy through using the immune system to eliminate a final common pathway of the malignant clone. However, significant hurdles remain in the generation of protein-specific immunity of sufficient magnitude effectively to prevent malignancy.

References

Aoki, T., Tashiro, K., Miyatake, S., Kinashi, T., Nakano, T., Oda, Y., Kikuchi, H. and Honjo, T. (1992). Expression of murine interleukin 7 in a murine glioma cell line results in reduced tumorigenicity in vivo. *Proceedings of the National Academy of Sciences of the United States of America*, **89**: 3850–4.

Arca, M. J., Krauss, J. C., Aruga, A., Cameron, M. J., Shu, S. and Chang, A. E. (1996). Therapeutic efficacy of T cells derived from lymph nodes draining a poorly immunogenic tumor transduced to secrete GM-CSF. *Cancer Gene Therapy*, **3**: 39–47.

Asher, A. L., Mule, J. J., Kasid, A., Restifo, N. P., Salo, J. C., Reichert, C. M., Jaffe, G., Fendly, B., Kriegler, M. and Rosenberg, S. A. (1991). Murine tumor cells transduced with the gene for tumor necrosis factor-α. *Journal of Immunology*, **146**: 3227–34.

Blankenstein, T., Qin, Z., Oberla, K., Müller, W., Rosen, H., Volk, H.-D. and Diamanstein, T. (1991). Tumor suppression after tumor cell-targeted tumor necrosis factor: a gene transfer. *Journal of Experimental Medicine*, **173**: 1047–52.

Chen, L., Ashe, S., Brady, W. A., Hellstrom, I., Hellstrom, K. E., Ledbetter, J. A., McGowan, P. and Linsley, P. S. (1992). Costimulation of antitumor immunity by the B7 counterreceptor for the T lymphocyte molecules CD28 and CTLA-4. *Cell*, **71**: 1093–102.

Chen, L., McGowan, P., Ashe, S., Johnston, J., Li, Y., Hellstrom, I. and Hellstrom, K. E. (1994). Tumor immunogenicity determines the effect of B7 costimulation on T cell-mediated tumor immunity. *Journal of Experimental Medicine*, **179**: 523–32.

Clements, V. K., Baskar, S., Armstrong, T. D. and Ostrand-Rosenberg, S. (1992). Invariant chain alters the malignant phenotype of MHC class II + tumor cells. *Journal of Immunology*, **149**: 2391–6.

Cole, G. A., Cole, G. A., Clements, V. K., Garcia, E. P. and Ostrand-Rosenberg, S. (1987). Allogenic H-2 antigen expression is insufficient for tumor rejection. *Proceedings of the National Academy of Sciences of the United States of America*, **84**: 8613–17.

Colombo, M. P., Ferrari, G., Stoppacciaro, A., Parenza, M., Rodolfo, M., Mavilio, F. and Parmiani, G. (1991). Granulocyte colony-stimulating factor gene transfer suppresses tumorigenicity of a murine adenocarcinoma in vivo. *Journal of Experimental Medicine*, **173**: 889–97.

Connor, J., Bannerji, R., Saito, S., Heston, W., Fair, W. and Gilboa, E. (1993). Regression of bladder tumors in mice treated with interleukin 2 gene-modified tumor cells. *Journal of Experimental Medicine*, **177**: 1127–34.

Dranoff, G., Jaffee, E., Lazenby, A., Golumbek, P., Levitsky, H., Brose, K., Jackson, V., Hamada, H., Pardoll, D. and Mulligan, R. C. (1993). Vaccination with irradiated tumor cells engineered to secrete murine granulocyte-macrophage colony-stimulating factor stimulates potent, specific, and long-lasting anti-tumor immunity. *Proceedings of the National Academy of Sciences of the United States of America*, **90**: 3539–43.

Esumi, N., Hunt, B., Itaya, T. and Frost, P. (1991). Reduced tumorigenicity of murine tumor cells secreting interferon is due to nonspecific host responses and is unrelated to class I major histocompatibility complex expression. *Cancer Research*, **51**: 1185–9.

Fearon, E. R., Pardoll, D. M., Itaya, T., Golumbek, P., Levitsky, H. I., Simons, J. W., Karasuyama, H., Vogelstein, B. and Frost, P. (1990). Interleukin-2 production by tumor cells bypasses T helper function in the generation of an antitumor response. *Cell*, **60**: 397–403.

Gansbacher, B., Zier, K., Daniels, B., Cronin, K., Bannerji, R. and Gilboa, E. (1990a). Interleukin 2 gene transfer into tumor cells abrogates tumorigenicity and induces protective immunity. *Journal of Experimental Medicine*, **172**: 1217–24.

Gansbacher, B., Bannerji, R., Daniels, B., Zier, K., Cronin, K. and Gilboa, E. (1990b). Retroviral vector-mediated-interferon gene transfer into tumor cells generates potent and long lasting antitumor immunity. *Cancer Research*, **50**: 7820–5.

Golumbek, P. T., Lazenby, A. J., Levitsky, H. I., Jaffee, L. M., Karasuyama, H., Baker, M. and Pardoll, D. M. (1991). Treatment of established renal cancer by tumor cells engineered to secrete interleukin-4. *Science*, **254**: 713–16.

Guo, Y., Wu, M., Chen, H., Wang, X., Liu, G., Li, G., Ma, J. and Sy, M.-S. (1994). Effective tumor vaccine generated by fusion of hepatoma cells with activated B cells. *Science*, **263**: 518–20.

Hock, H., Dorsch, M., Diamantstein, T. and Blankenstein, T. (1991). Interleukin 7 induces CD4 T cell-dependent tumor rejection. *Journal of Experimental Medicine*, **174**: 1291–8.

Hock, H., Dorsch, M., Kunzendorf, U., Oberla, K., Qin, Z., Diamantstein, T. and Blankenstein, T. (1993a). Vaccinations with tumor cells genetically engineered to produce different cytokines: Effectively not superior to a classical adjuvant. *Cancer Research*, **53**: 714–16.

Hock, H., Dorsch, M., Kunzendorf, U., Qin, Z., Diamantstein, T. and Blankenstein, T. (1993b). Mechanisms of rejection induced by tumor cell-targeted gene transfer of interleukin 2, interleukin 4, interleukin 7, tumor necrosis factor, or interferon. *Proceedings of the National Academy of Sciences of the United States of America*, **90**: 2774–8.

Hui, K., Grosveld, F. and Festenstein, H. (1984). Rejection of transplantable AKR leukaemia cells following MHC DNA-mediated cell transformation. *Nature*, **311**: 750–52.

Kawakami, Y., Rosenberg, S. A. and Lotze, M. T. (1988). Interleukin 4 promotes the growth of tumor-infiltrating lymphocytes cytotoxic for human autologous melanoma. *Journal of Experimental Medicine*, **168**: 2183–91.

Krauss, J. C., Strome, S. E., Chang, A. E. and Shu, S. (1994). Generation of therapeutic

T cells from lymph nodes draining a tumor genetically engineered to secrete interleukin 4. *Journal of Cell Biology*, **18A**: 242.

Kroemer, G., Andreu, J. L., Gonzalo, J. A., Gutierrez-Ramos, J. C., Martinez, A. C. (1991). Interleukin-2, autotolerance, and autoimmunity. *Advances in Immunology*, **50**: 147–235.

Lukacs, K. V., Lowrie, D. B., Sokes, R. W. and Colston, M. J. (1993). Tumor cells transfected with a bacterial heat-shock gene lose tumorigenicity and induce protection against tumors. *Journal of Experimental Medicine*, **178**: 343–8.

McBride, W. H., Thacker, J. D., Comora, S., Economou, J. S., Kelley, D., Hogge, D., Dubinett, S. M. and Dougherty, G. J. (1992). Genetic modification of a murine fibrosarcoma to produce interleukin 7 stimulates host cell infiltration and tumor immunity. *Cancer Research*, **52**: 3931–7.

Mulé, J. J., Yang, J. C., Lafreniere, R. L., Shu, S. and Rosenberg, S. A. (1987). Identification of cellular mechanisms operational in vivo during the regression of established pulmonary metastases by the systemic administration of high-dose recombinant interleukin 2. *Journal of Immunology*, **139**: 285–94.

Mullen, C. A., Coale, M. M., Levy, A. T., Stetler-Stevenson, W. G., Liotta, L. A., Brandt, S. and Blease, R. M. (1992). Fibrosarcoma cells transduced with the IL-6 gene exhibit reduced tumorigenicity, increased immunogenicity, and decreased metastatic potential. *Cancer Research*, **52**: 6020–4.

Nabel, G. J., Nabel, E. G., Yang, Z., Fox, B. A., Plautz, G. E., Gao, X., Huang, L., Shu, S., Gordon, D. and Chang, A. E. (1993). Direct gene transfer with DNA–liposome complexes in melanoma: Expression, biologic activity, and lack of toxicity in humans. *Proceedings of the National Academy of Sciences of the United States of America*, **90**: 11307–11.

Oliff, A., Defeo-Jones, D., Boyer, M., Martinez, D., Kiefer, D., Vuocolo, G., Wolfe, A. and Socher, S. H. (1987). Tumors secreting human TNF/Cachectin induce cachexia in mice. *Cell*, **50**: 555–63.

Ostrand-Rosenberg, S., Thakur, A. and Clements, V. (1990). Rejection of mouse sarcoma cells after transfection of MHC class II genes. *Journal of Immunology*, **144**: 4068–71.

Ostrand-Rosenberg, S., Roby, C. A. and Clements, V. K. (1991). Abrogation of tumorigenicity by MHC Class II antigen expression requires the cytoplasmic domain of the Class II molecule. *Journal of Immunology*, **147**: 2419–22.

Plautz, G. E., Yang, Z., Wu, B., Gao, X., Huang, L. and Nabel, G. J. (1993). Immunotherapy of malignancy by in vivo gene transfers into tumors. *Proceedings of the National Academy of Sciences of the United States of America*, **90**: 4645–9.

Porgador, A., Tzehoval, E., Katz, A., Vadai, E., Revel, M., Feldman, M. and Eisenbach, L. (1992). Interleukin 6 gene transfer into Lewis lung carcinoma tumor cells suppresses the malignant phenotype and confers immunotherapeutic competence against parental metastatic cells. *Cancer Research*, **52**: 3679–86.

Porgador, A., Bannerji, R., Watanabe, Y., Feldman, M., Gilboa, E. and Eisenbach, L. (1993). Antimetastatic vaccination of tumor-bearing mice with two types of IFN-gene-inserted tumor cells. *Journal of Immunology*, **150**: 1458–70.

Restifo, N. P., Spiess, P. J., Karp, S. E., Mulé, J. J. and Rosenberg, S. A. (1992). A nonimmunogenic sarcoma transduced with the cDNA for interferon elicits CD8 T cells against the wild-type tumor: Correlation with antigen presentation capability. *Journal of Experimental Medicine*, **175**: 1423–31.

Rosenberg, S. A., Lotze, M. T., Muul, L. M. et al. (1985). Observations on the systemic administration of autologous lymphokine-activated killer cells and recombinant interleukin-2 to patients with metastatic cancer. *New England Journal of Medicine*, **313**: 1485–92.

Schwartz, R. H. (1992). Costimulation of T lymphocytes: The role of CD28, CTLA-4, and B7/BB1 in interleukin-2 production and immunotherapy. *Cell*, 71: 1065–8.

Shawler, D. L., Dorigo, O., Gjerset, R. A., Royston, I., Sobol, R. E. and Fakhrai, H. (1995). Comparison of gene therapy with interleukin-2 gene modified fibroblasts and tumor cells in the murine CT-26 models of colorectal carcinoma. *Journal of Immunotherapy*, 17: 201–8.

Stoppacciaro, A., Melani, C., Parenza, M., Mastracchio, A., Bassi, C., Baroni, C., Parmiani, G. and Colombo, M. P. (1993). Regression of an established tumor genetically modified to release granulocyte colony-stimulating factor requires granulocyte-T cell cooperation and T cell-produced interferon-γ. *Journal of Experimental Medicine*, 178: 151–61.

Swain, S. L. (1991). Lymphokines and the immune response: the central role of interleukin-2. *Current Opinion in Immunology*, 3: 304–10.

Tahara, H., Zitvogel, L., Storkus, W. J., Zeh II, H. J., McKinney, T. G., Schreiber, R. D., Gubler, U., Robbins, P. D. and Lotze, M. T. (1995). Effective eradication of established murine tumors with IL-12 gene therapy using a polycistronic retroviral vector. *Journal of Immunology*, 154: 6466–74.

Tanaka, K., Isselbacher, K. J., Khoury, G. and Jay, G. (1985). Reversal of oncogenesis by the expression of a major histocompatibility complex class I gene. *Science*, 228: 26–30.

Tanaka, K., Gorelik, E., Watanabe, M., Hozumi, N. and Jay, G. (1988). Rejection of B16 melanoma induced by expression of a transfected major histocompatibility complex class I gene. *Molecular and Cellular Biology*, 8: 1857–61.

Teng, M. N., Park, B. H., Koeppen, H. K. W., Tracey, K. J., Fendly, B. M. and Schreiber, H. (1991). Long-term inhibition of tumor growth by tumor necrosis factor in the absence of cachexia or T-cell immunity. *Proceedings of the National Academy of Sciences of the United States of America*, 88: 3535–9.

Tepper, R. I., Coffman, R. L. and Leder, P. (1992).An eosinophil-dependent mechanism for the antitumor effect of interleukin-4. *Science*, 257: 548–51.

Tepper, R. I., Levinson, D. A., Stanger, B. Z., Campos-Torres, J., Abbas, A. K. and Leder, P. (1990). IL-4 induces allergic-like inflammatory disease and alters T cell development in transgenic mice. *Cell*, 62: 457–67.

Tepper, R. I., Pattengale, P. K. and Leder, P. (1989). Murine interleukin-4 displays potent anti-tumor activity in vivo. *Cell*, 57: 503–12.

Townsend, S. E. and Allison, J. P. (1993). Tumor rejection after direct costimulation of CD8+ T cells by B7-transfected melanoma cells. *Science*, 259: 368–70.

Wallich, R., Bulbuc, N., Hammerling, G. J., Katzav, S., Segal, S. and Feldman, M. (1985). Abrogation of metastatic properties of tumor cells by de novo expression of H-2K antigens following H-2 gene transfection. *Nature*, 315: 301–5.

Watanabe, Y., Kuribayashi, K., Miyatake, S., Nishihara, K., Nakayama, E., Taniyama, T. and Sakata, T. (1989). Exogenous expression of mouse interferon-cDNA in mouse neuroblastoma C1300 cells results in reduced tumorigenicity by augmented anti-tumor immunity. *Proceedings of the National Academy of Sciences of the United States of America*, 86: 9456–60.

7

Genetically modified lymphocytes and hematopoietic stem cells as therapeutic vehicles

PATRICK J. GERAGHTY AND JAMES J. MULÉ

Introduction

The application of efficient gene-transfer techniques to lymphocyte populations has opened new pathways in the therapy of neoplastic disease. Genetically engineered lymphocytes possess unique functional characteristics which can be exploited in novel treatment protocols. The ability of lymphocytes to traffic to tumor deposits can be harnessed to effect the delivery of therapeutically active molecules to the tumor microenvironment. Specific changes in the local tumor milieu may augment the host immune response, while avoiding the toxicity associated with high-dose systemic administration of cytokines. In addition, the construction of chimeric T cell receptors has led to the direct coupling of the recognition and effector phases of the immune response. In addition, advances in the isolation and propagation of specific hematopoietic stem cell (HSC) populations may enable researchers partially to reconstitute the hematolymphoid system with genetically engineered precursor cells possessing specific antitumor activity. Targeting of HSC may allow the indirect transfer of genes into lymphocytic effector populations, while overcoming some of the limitations associated with direct gene insertion into mature lymphocytes. This chapter reviews methods of gene transfer into lymphocytes and HSC and the in-vivo characteristics of these cells following adoptive transfer. Strategies for using genetic modification of lymphocytes and HSC to enhance the antitumor immune response are discussed, and the relative merits of using either the mature lymphocyte or HSC populations for gene therapy of cancer are examined.

Methods of gene transfer into mature lymphocytes and hematopoietic stem cells

Several factors must be considered in selecting an appropriate technique of gene transfer. As most patients qualifying for these therapeutic approaches have disseminated malignancies, their diminished physiologic reserves limit the applicability of time-consuming methods used to select cloned lymphocyte lines expressing the desired gene. While evidence is mounting for the conserved use of T cell receptor (TCR) rearrangement sequences in the antitumor response, harvested tumor-infiltrating lymphocytes or tumor-draining lymph node cells represent heterogeneous populations which probably contain polyclonal tumor-reactive populations. Therefore, use of low-efficiency transfection techniques followed by negative selection of transfected cells may result in unfavorable restriction of the T cell repertoire, limiting the effective immune response. Similar caveats apply to gene transfer into harvested HSC populations. These factors would rule out the use of most nonviral methods of gene transfer, such as lipid-based transfection, calcium phosphate coprecipitation, and electroporation. Particle-mediated gene transfer does show promise for applications requiring stably transfected lymphocytes, as this method has been shown in some studies to mediate gene integration with efficiency comparable to retroviral vectors (Woffendin et al., 1994). However, use of such a mode of direct gene insertion for successful transfection of HSC has not been reported to date.

Therefore, efficient gene transfer into bulk populations of harvested lymphocytes or HSC would most reliably be performed by virally mediated gene delivery. A variety of viral vectors is currently available for such purposes, and the favorable and unfavorable characteristics of each vector will help determine its applicability to a given therapeutic strategy (Miller, 1992; Morgan, Tompkins and Yarmush, 1993; Jolly, 1994; Berns and Giraud, 1995; Haddada, Cordier and Perricaudet, 1995).

Retroviral vectors

Modified retroviruses, along with adeno-associated viruses, are the only vectors which integrate into the mammalian genome following cellular entry. Host genome integration ensures that the transduced gene(s) will be heritably transmitted to subsequent cellular generations – an invaluable mechanism in strategies which aim to introduce a resident population of tumor-reactive lymphocytes or HSC. Transduction of actively replicating target cells is relatively efficient; however, host transcriptional regulation may lead to relatively low expression of the introduced gene (Hwu et al., 1993b).

Deletion of structural genes renders these vectors replication incompetent, and the protein products necessary for assembly of infectious virions are supplied *in trans* by the packaging cell line. In one early experiment, T-cell lymphomas were reported in primates following recombinant events which led to the generation of replication-competent virus (Donahue et al., 1992). Subsequent manipulations of the viral backbone and development of sensitive screening techniques for the presence of replication-competent virus in packaging cell line supernatants have minimized the risk of further similar mishaps. Extensive experience with retrovirally transduced cells in carefully monitored human trials has accumulated, and no sequelae of untoward recombinant events have been reported, to date.

Adenoviral and pox viral vectors

Unlike retroviral vectors, modified adenovirus and pox virus vectors do not readily integrate into the host genome, and expression of the transferred gene is therefore transient. Advantageous aspects of these vectors include the ability to transfect nondividing cells, and a greater efficiency of transfection than retroviruses. Pox viruses (fowlpox, vaccinia) also encode a native transcriptional assemblage, freeing them from host transcriptional control. Further data on the safety of these vectors in human subjects are needed, but their ability to provide brief, high-level expression of the transferred gene may find a role in appropriate protocols.

In-vivo characteristics of transferred lymphocytes and hematopoietic stem cells

Over the past two decades intensive research efforts have garnered much information concerning the in-vivo distribution, lifespan, and toxicity of adoptively transferred immune lymphocytes. Early studies addressed these questions using radiolabeled tumor infiltrating lymphocytes (TIL), and showed that TIL preferentially trafficked to tumor deposits to a greater degree than did transferred peripheral blood lymphocytes (PBL) (Fisher et al., 1989; Griffith et al., 1989; Pockaj et al., 1994). Localization to tumor sites correlated with the ability of TIL to effect in-vivo antitumor responses, and generated interest in the use of gene-modified TIL to enhance antitumor immunity via changes in the tumor microenvironment and/or the functional characteristics of the TIL themselves.

More recent efforts have employed gene-marking techniques to answer similar questions regarding the fate of adoptively transferred, gene-modified TIL. Gene-marking strategies offer a dual advantage. First, retroviral transduction of transferred lymphocytes allows for improved detection of the progeny of the infused cells. Whereas cellular isotope concentrations are decreased by each cell division, copy number of the integrated marker gene (usually a selectable gene such as the neomycin resistance gene, neo^R) is not diminished in subsequent lymphocyte generations. Molecular biology techniques allow for increased sensitivity in the detection of the gene-modified lymphocytes, including their recovery by ex-vivo culture in selection media (Kasid et al., 1990; Rosenberg et al., 1990; Favrot and Philip, 1992). Additionally, researchers simultaneously generate information on the safety profile of retrovirally transduced lymphocytes.

In 1990, Rosenberg et al. reported the results of a landmark study in which five patients with metastatic melanoma were treated with systemic IL-2 administration and adoptive transfer of TIL that had been transduced with the neo^R gene. Using polymerase chain reaction techniques, they documented the presence of modified TIL in peripheral blood and tumor deposits for up to 60 days postinfusion. Three of the five patients experienced partial or complete responses following therapy, and no ill-effects attributable to the transfer of retrovirally modified cells were reported. Accompanying in-vitro studies of the transduced lymphocytes showed no alterations in growth pattern, TCR gene rearrangement usage, or IL-2 dependence when compared to unmodified syngeneic TIL (Kasid et al., 1990). Taken together, these studies provided support for the use of genetically engineered lymphocytes for the treatment of cancer.

Similar gene-marking studies have been used to investigate the in-vivo characteristics of transferred pluripotent stem cells. In recipients of neo^R-transduced autologous bone marrow transplants, the marker gene was expressed in all hematopoietic lineages for at least 18 months, indicative of both successful stem cell retroviral transduction (at efficiency rates of 5%) and successful in-vivo engraftment of the transduced cells (Brenner et al., 1993). More concrete evidence of successful pluripotent stem cell transduction was recently offered by Nolta et al. (1996), who transduced human CD34+ progenitor cells with a retroviral vector prior to engraftment in immuno-deficient recipient mice. Analysis of the murine bone marrow seven months later demonstrated integration of the retroviral vector at identical sites in human myeloid and lymphoid cells, proving descent from a transduced HSC precursor. Again, no toxicity specifically attributable to the gene-modified cells was reported. Long-term survival of transduced HSC has favorable implications for the possible use of these cells for gene therapy of cancer.

Cautionary notes have been sounded, however. A more recent gene-marking trial examining the activities of transferred TIL versus PBL failed to demonstrate an advantage of TIL in concentrating at the tumor sites (Economou et al., 1996). However, in this study, evidence was not provided that the transferred TIL showed specific and autologous antitumor reactivity in vitro prior to systemic administration to the patients. Thus, it is possible that the lack of homing to tumor sites was the result of insufficient tumor specificity in the transferred TIL. Additionally, a recent trial of HIV-seropositive patients who received adoptive transfer of *gag*-specific cytotoxic T lymphocytes (CTL) that had been retrovirally transduced with the hygromycin phosphotransferase (Hy) and thymidine kinase (TK) suicide genes provided evidence concerning the potential difficulties of maintaining viable populations of modified lymphocytes. The trial demonstrated that even severely immunocompromised individuals can mount CTL responses against the antigenic determinants of foreign genes (Hy and TK), effectively clearing the transferred cells from the circulation (Riddell et al., 1996). This finding suggests potential negative consequences for the use of genetically modified lymphocytes and HSC in patients who have not received prior complete myeloablative therapy.

Strategies for genetic modification of lymphocytes and hematopoietic stem cells

Successful gene transfer into lymphocytes and HSC allows the researcher to envision a wide range of novel applications of this technique to cancer immunotherapy. A logical method of designing new approaches would begin with an examination of the shortcomings of current adoptive immunotherapy techniques. After areas in need of improvement have been specified, genes that may improve the efficacy or reduce the toxicity of treatment may be selected for testing. Table 7.1 outlines such an approach, and provides a partial listing of active and proposed protocols. Several of the approaches which have been investigated in animal models and human trials are discussed below.

Interleukin 2

Interleukin 2 (IL-2) is a T cell growth factor. Treatment of patients with disseminated melanoma with systemic, high-dose IL-2 therapy alone results in a small percentage of clinical responses, but is accompanied by substantial toxicity (Rosenberg et al., 1989). In a similar fashion, clinical responses following adoptive transfer of TIL are dependent upon the concomitant administration of exogenous IL-2.

Table 7.1. *Potential directions for genetic modification of adoptively transferred lymphocytes and hematopoietic stem cells*

Desired alteration	Genes of interest
Reduce systemic administration of toxic cytokines (i.e., IL-2, TNF-α) through local cytokine production in the tumor microenvironment following homing of the transferred lymphocytes	IL-2, IL-2 receptor TNF-α GM-CSF
Prolong lifespan of transferred cells	IL-2, IL-2 receptor Protein kinase C-γ
Enable in-vivo selection of transferred cells	Multidrug resistance 1 (*MDR*1)
Enable in-vivo eradication of transferred cells	Thymidine kinase Cytosine deaminase Hygromycin phosphotransferase
Redirect TCR repertoire to defined tumor antigens	Chimeric TCR TCRα and TCRβ
Escape MHC restriction of T cell response	Chimeric TCR
Attract defined effector cell subsets to tumor site	Chemokines
Enhance effector cell trafficking to tumor site	Chemokine receptors

Gene therapy that would render TIL independent of exogenous IL-2 would clearly be advantageous. Previous experiments investigating a role for IL-2 autocrine overstimulation in the development of T cell lymphomas have demonstrated that T cells transfected with the IL-2 gene proliferate in the absence of exogenous IL-2, and form tumors in nude mice (Yamada et al., 1987; Karasuyama, Tohyama and Tada, 1989). Subsequently, Nakamura et al. (1994) conducted an adoptive immunotherapy trial in which metastatic murine melanomas were treated with either unmodified TIL or TIL that had been retrovirally transduced with the gene for IL-2. The gene-modified TIL were significantly more effective in eradicating metastatic disease than were the unmodified TIL.

Tumor necrosis factor-α

Tumor necrosis factor-α (TNF-α) has been shown to mediate regression of tumors when given intralesionally (Bartsch et al., 1989) or via isolated limb perfusion (Thom et al., 1995), but cannot be administered systemically in therapeutic doses due to toxicity (Sherman et al., 1988). Hwu et al. (1993b) have transduced TIL with the gene for TNF-α, with the intent that as the TIL localize to tumor deposits, the introduced transgene will generate enough local production of the cytokine to mediate tumor killing, while reducing or eliminating the potential of systemic side-effects. Initial production of secreted TNF-α by the transduced TIL was low, necessitating modification of the transgene to eliminate the membrane-bound form of the cytokine and enhance production of the secreted form. Truncation of the transmembrane domain of the cytokine, which prevented binding to the endoplasmic reticulum, resulted in the fivefold increase in the secreted form of TNF-α. Human trials with these transduced TIL are currently under way.

Protein kinase C-γ

In addition to exogenous IL-2, maintenance of antigen-specific TIL populations in vitro requires periodic stimulation with antigen. As protein kinase C-γ (PKC-γ) is a downstream effector in the TCR pathway response to antigen, Finn et al. (1991) examined the effects of retroviral transduction of PKC-γ into TIL. The transduced cells were able to be maintained in long-term culture without antigen stimulation; however, antigen specificity identical to that of the parental cells was preserved.

Multidrug resistance 1 and heat stable antigen

The multidrug resistance 1 gene (*MDR-1*) confers resistance to several chemotherapeutic agents, including taxol. Sorrentino et al. (1992) demonstrated that murine HSC retrovirally transduced with the *MDR-1* gene prior to transplant into donor mice could subsequently be selected for in vivo by administration of taxol. In future applications to cancer immunotherapy, transferred HSC which have been double transduced – with both *MDR-1* and a gene conferring enhanced antitumor activity – could subsequently be selectively enriched for relative to the native bone marrow. Alternatively Medin et al. (1996) have recently described transduction of CD34+ cells with a bicistronic retroviral vector encoding both therapeutic (glucocerebrosidase) and selectable (heat stable antigen, HSA) genes. The transduced fraction can be sorted on the basis of cell surface expression of HSA prior to transfer, and 100% pure populations of transduced HSC can be generated. Thus, methods exist for the selection of transduced HSC both prior to and after therapeutic transfer.

Chimeric T cell receptors

Kuwana and coworkers first reported the combination of immunoglobulin-derived variable regions possessing specificity for tumor antigens and T cell receptor constant regions to form a chimeric TCR (Kuwana et al., 1987).

This construct required transfection of two separate genes in order to form a functional TCRα–TCRβ complex. Subsequently, Eshhar et al. (1993) demonstrated a modified chimeric TCR in which a single-chain variable domain from the antibody is directly coupled to the γ or ζ transduction subunits of the TCR. This chimeric TCR construct can be encoded on a single gene, facilitating the transfection of the desired effector cells. They showed that the complex was expressed as a functional surface group on transfected CTL, and that binding to the specific antigen resulted in IL-2 secretion and non-major histocompatibility (MHC)-restricted lysis of target cells. The lack of MHC restriction is due to the fact that this construct recognizes antibody-defined antigens, rather than peptides within the MHC groove.

Chimeric TCR represents a potentially powerful tool for tumor therapy. Stancovski et al. (1993) transfected CTL with the gene encoding a single-chain chimeric TCR gene with specificity for Neu/HER2, a known breast carcinoma-associated antigen. These modified CTL demonstrated specific recognition and lysis of target cells expressing Neu/HER2. In a similar fashion, Hwu et al. (1993a) utilized TIL transduced with a chimeric TCR construct possessing specificity for a defined ovarian cancer antigen to achieve specific cytolytic activity against cells expressing the target antigen.

While the above experiments utilized TIL as vehicles, transduction of similar genes into HSC could 'skew' the T cell repertoire to target residual disease following autologous bone marrow or peripheral blood stem cell transplants. Presumably, genes under the appropriate control of tissue-specific or cell-specific promoters/enhancers could render daughter lymphocytes and/or monocytes tumor reactive through expression of the transgene-encoded chimeric TCR.

It must be emphasized that the above examples represent only a partial sampling of the various gene modifications which can be performed to enhance adoptive immunotherapy of cancer. Gene therapy of cancer remains in its infancy, however, and new avenues of research will no doubt proliferate in the coming years.

Choosing a cellular vehicle: mature lymphocytes versus stem cells

To date, the majority of adoptive immunotherapy models have utilized mature T lymphocytes (TIL or PBL) as effector cells. In addition, as gene therapy protocols have been examined (see Table 7.1), most have utilized mature lymphocytes. Factors contributing to the use of these cells include their relative ease of harvest and ability to traffic to tumor deposits.

However, as research in the arena of gene therapy expands, a reassessment

Table 7.2. *Choosing a cell for genetic modification: advantages and disadvantages of mature lymphocytes versus hematopoietic stem cells*

Advantages	Disadvantages
Lymphocytes	
Previous sensitization to tumor antigens	Surgical resection needed for harvest
Ability to traffic to tumor sites	Need for ex-vivo expansion
	Altered phenotype secondary to ex-vivo expansion
	Finite lifespan
	Low efficiency of gene transfer
	Poor expression of transgene
Hematopoietic stem cells	
High gene transfer efficiency unnecessary as only partial reconstitution of marrow is needed	Myelosuppression necessary prior to HSC transplant
Ex-vivo expansion not required as cells undergo in-vivo expansion	Unknown if T cell progeny effectively traffic to tumor sites
Ease of harvest from G-CSF-mobilized peripheral blood	
Multilineage differentiation	
Self-renewing	
Unlimited lifespan	

of the choice of targeted vehicles is necessary. Table 7.2 outlines several pros and cons associated with the use of either cellular vehicle. Specifically, the use of transduced HSC in these protocols would ensure that a self-renewing population of tumor-reactive immune cells would be established in the patient, providing a 'one-time, long-lasting' therapeutic approach. Mature lymphocytes have a finite lifespan, and tumor which is not fully eradicated prior to the end of that period may escape the adoptive immune response.

In addition, the use of HSC may reduce the need for truly high-efficiency transduction of the transferred cells. Whereas high rates of transduction are needed to achieve active levels of gene expression in mature lymphocytes, relatively small numbers of transduced, engrafted HSC can subsequently undergo substantial in-vivo expansion, giving rise to therapeutic populations of effector cells.

Conclusion

Genetically modified lymphocytes and hematopoietic stem cells show great promise for use as therapeutic vehicles in gene therapy of cancer. These modified cellular populations may enable researchers to limit the toxicity associated with previous adoptive immunotherapy protocols, yet simultaneously enhance the antitumor activity of the transferred cells.

Early laboratory and clinical trials utilizing a variety of transgenes have shown that dependence on systemic cytokine administration can be reduced, recognition of tumor antigens can be enhanced, and selection of the effector cell populations prior to or following transfer to the host can be accomplished.

The use of genetically engineered hematopoietic stem cells for cancer therapy represents a particularly exciting area of investigation. The pluripotent, self-renewing nature of these cells may enable researchers to establish long-lasting, multilineage cellular populations which have been genetically modified to show specific antitumor activity, and thus may provide a valuable new weapon in the armamentarium of the clinical oncologist.

References

Bartsch, H., Pfizenmaier, K., Schroeder, M. and Nagel, G. (1989). Intralesional application of recombinant human tumor necrosis factor alpha induces local tumor regression in patients with advanced malignancies. *European Journal of Cancer and Clinical Oncology*, **25**: 287.

Berns, K. I. and Giraud, C. (1995). Adenovirus and adeno-associated virus as vectors for gene therapy. *Annals of the New York Academy of Science*, **772**: 95.

Brenner, M. K., Rill, D. R., Holladay, M. S., Heslop, H. E., Moen, R. C., Buschle, M., Krance, R. A., Santana, V. M., Anderson, W. F. and Ihle, J. N. (1993). Gene marking to determine whether autologous marrow infusion restored long-term haemopoiesis in cancer patients. *Lancet*, **342**: 1134.

Donahue, R. E., Kessler, S. W., Bodine, D., McDonagh, K., Dunbar, C., Goodman, S., Agricola, B., Byrne, E., Raffeld, M., Moen, R., Bacher, J., Zesbo, K. M. and Nienhuis, A. W. (1992). Helper virus induced T cell lymphoma in nonhuman primates after retroviral mediated gene transfer. *Journal of Experimental Medicine*, **176**: 1125.

Economou, J. S., Belldegrun, A. S., Glaspy, J., Toloza, E. M., Figlin, R., Hobbs, J., Meldon, N., Kaboo, R., Tso, C. L., Miller, A., Lau, R., McBride, W. and Moen, R. C. (1996). In vivo trafficking of adoptively transferred interleukin-2 expanded tumor-infiltrating lymphocytes and peripheral blood lymphocytes: results of a double gene marking trial. *Journal of Clinical Investigation*, **97**: 515.

Eshhar, Z., Waks, T., Gross, G. and Schindler, D. G. (1993). Specific activation and targeting of cytotoxic lymphocytes through chimeric single chains consisting of antibody-binding domains and the γ or ζ subunits of the immunoglobulin and T-cell receptors. *Proceedings of the National Academy of Sciences of the United States of America*, **90**: 720.

Favrot, M. C. and Philip, T. (1992). Treatment of patients with advanced cancer using tumor infiltrating lymphocytes transduced with the gene of resistance to neomycin. *Human Gene Therapy*, **3**: 533.

Finn, O. J., Persons, D. A., Bendt, K. M., Pirami, L. and Ricciardi, P. (1991). Retroviral transduction of protein kinase C-γ into cytotoxic T lymphocyte clones leads to immortalization with retention of specific function. *Journal of Immunology*, **146**: 1099.

Fisher, B., Packard, B. S., Read, E. J., Carrasquillo, J. A., Carter, C. S., Topalian, S. L., Yang, J. C., Yolles, P., Larson, S. M. and Rosenberg, S. A. (1989). Tumor localization of adoptively transferred indium-111 labeled tumor infiltrating lymphocytes in patients with metastatic melanoma. *Journal of Clinical Oncology*, 7: 250.

Griffith, K. D., Read, E. J., Carrasquillo, J. A., Carter, C. S., Yang, J. C., Fisher, B., Aebersold, P., Packard, B. S., Yu, M. Y. and Rosenberg, S. A. (1989). In vivo distribution of adoptively transferred indium-111-labeled tumor infiltrating lymphocytes and peripheral blood lymphocytes in patients with metastatic melanoma. *Journal of the National Cancer Institute*, 81: 1709.

Haddada, H., Cordier, L. and Perricaudet, M. (1995). Gene therapy using adenovirus vectors. *Current Topics in Microbiology and Immunology*, 199(Pt 3): 297.

Hwu, P., Shafer, G. E., Treisman, J., Schindler, D. G., Gross, G., Cowherd, R., Rosenberg, S. A. and Eshhar, Z. (1993a). Lysis of ovarian cancer cells by human lymphocytes redirected with a chimeric gene composed of an antibody variable region and the Fc receptor γ chain. *Journal of Experimental Medicine*, 178: 361.

Hwu, P., Yannelli, J., Kriegler, M., Anderson, W. F., Perez, C., Chiang, Y., Schwarz, S., Cowherd, R., Delgado, C., Mulé, J. and Rosenberg, S. A. (1993b). Functional and molecular characterization of tumor-infiltrating lymphocytes transduced with tumor necrosis factor-α cDNA for the gene therapy of cancer in humans. *Journal of Immunology*, 150: 4104.

Jolly, D. (1994). Viral vector systems for gene therapy. *Cancer Gene Therapy*, 1: 51.

Karasuyama, H., Tohyama, N. and Tada, T. (1989). Autocrine growth and tumorigenicity of interleukin-2 dependent helper T cells transfected with the IL-2 gene. *Journal of Experimental Medicine*, 169: 13.

Kasid, A., Morecki, S., Aebersold, P., Cornetta, K., Culver, K., Freeman, S., Director, E., Lotze, M. T., Blaese, R. M., Anderson, W. F. and Rosenberg, S. A. (1990). Human gene transfer: characterization of human tumor-infiltrating lymphocytes as vehicles for retroviral-mediated gene transfer in man. *Proceedings of the National Academy of Sciences of the United States of America*, 87: 473.

Kuwana, Y., Asakura, Y., Utsunomiya, N., Nakanishi, M., Arata, Y., Itoh, S., Nagase, F. and Kurosawa, Y. (1987). Expression of chimeric receptor composed of immunoglobulin-derived V regions and T-cell receptor derived C regions. *Biochemical and Biophysical Research Communications*, 149: 960.

Medin, J. A., Migita, M., Pawliuk, R., Jacobson, S., Amiri, M., Luepfel-Stahl, S., Brady, R. O., Humphries, R. K. and Karlsson, S. (1996). A bicistronic therapeutic retroviral vector enables sorting of transduced CD34+ cells and corrects the enzyme deficiency in cells from Gaucher patients. *Blood,* 87: 1754.

Miller, A. D. (1992). Retroviral vectors. *Current Topics in Microbiology and Immunology*, 158: 1.

Morgan, J. R., Tompkins, R. G. and Yarmush, M. L. (1993). Advances in recombinant retroviruses for gene delivery. *Advanced Drug Delivery Reviews*, 12: 143.

Nakamura, Y., Wakimoto, H., Abe, J., Kanegae, Y., Saito, I., Aoyagi, M., Hirakawa, K. and Hamada, H. (1994). Adoptive immunotherapy with murine tumor-specific T lymphocytes engineered to secrete interleukin 2. *Cancer Research*, 54: 5757.

Nolta, J. A., Dao, M. A., Wells, S., Smogorzewska, E. M. and Kohn, D. B. (1996). Transduction of pluripotent human hematopoietic stem cells demonstrated by clonal analysis after engraftment in immune-deficient mice. *Proceedings of the National Academy of Sciences of the United States of America*, 93: 2414.

Pockaj, B. A., Sherry, R. M., Wei, J. P., Yannelli, J. R., Carter, C. S., Leitman, S. F., Carrasquillo, J. A., Steinberg, S. M., Rosenberg, S. A. and Yang, J. C. (1994).

Localization of 111-indium-labeled tumor infiltrating lymphocytes to tumor in patients receiving adoptive immunotherapy. *Cancer*, 73: 1731.

Riddell, S. R., Elliott, M., Lewinsohn, D. A., Gilbert, M. J., Wilson, L., Manley, S. A., Lupton, S. D., Overell, R. W., Reynolds, T. C., Corey, L. and Greenberg, P. D. (1996). T-cell mediated rejection of gene-modified HIV-specific cytotoxic T lymphocytes in HIV-infected patients. *Nature Medicine*, 2: 216.

Rosenberg, S. A., Lotze, M., Yang, J., Aebersold, P., Linehan, W. M., Seipp, C. and White, D. (1989). Experience with the use of high-dose interleukin-2 in the treatment of 652 cancer patients. *Annals of Surgery*, 210: 474.

Rosenberg, S. A., Aebersold, P., Cornetta, K., Kasid, A., Morgan, R. A., Moen, R., Karson, E. M., Lotze, M. T., Yang, J. C., Topalian, S. L., Merino, M. J., Culver, K., Miller, A. D., Blaese, R. M. and Anderson, W. F. (1990). Gene transfer into humans – immunotherapy of patients with advanced melanoma, using tumor-infiltrating lymphocytes modified by retroviral gene transduction. *New England Journal of Medicine*, 323: 570.

Sherman, M., Spriggs, D., Arthur, K., Imamura, K., Frei, E. and Kufe, D. (1988). Recombinant human tumor necrosis factor administered as a five-day continuous infusion in cancer patients: phase I toxicity and effects on lipid metabolism. *Journal of Clinical Oncology*, 6: 344.

Sorrentino, B. P., Brandt, S. J., Bodine, D., Gottesman, M., Pastan, I., Cline, A. and Nienhuis, A. W. (1992). Selection of drug-resistant bone marrow cells in vivo after retroviral transfer of human *MDR* 1. *Science*, 257: 99.

Stancovski, I., Schindler, D. G., Waks, T., Yarden, Y., Sela, M. and Eshhar, Z. (1993). Targeting of T lymphocytes to Neu/HER2-expressing cells using chimeric single chain Fv receptors. *Journal of Immunology*, 151: 6577.

Thom, A. K., Alexander, H. R., Andrich, M. P., Barker, W. C., Rosenberg, S. A. and Fraker, D. L. (1995). Cytokine levels and systemic toxicity in patients undergoing isolated limb perfusion with high-dose tumor necrosis factor, interferon gamma, and melphalan. *Journal of Clinical Oncology*, 13: 264.

Woffendin, C., Yang, Z-Y., Udaykumar, Xu, L., Yang, N-S., Sheehy, M. J. and Nabel, G. J. (1994). Nonviral and viral delivery of a human immunodeficiency virus protective gene into primary human T cells. *Proceedings of the National Academy of Sciences of the United States of America*, 91: 11581.

Yamada, G., Kitamura, Y., Sonoda, H., Harada, H., Taki, S., Mulligan, R. C., Osawa, H., Diamantstein, T., Yokoyama, S. and Taniguchi, T. (1987). Retroviral expression of the human IL-2 gene in a murine T cell line results in cell growth autonomy and tumorigenicity. *EMBO Journal*, 6: 2705.

8

Pharmacologic effects of oligonucleotides and some clinical applications

LEONARD M. NECKERS AND KANAK IYER

Introduction

Antisense RNA and DNA techniques have been developed as a relatively recent approach to the specific modulation of gene expression. The development of antisense RNA techniques began with observations from the laboratories of J. Tomizawa and N. Kleckner that bacteria can regulate gene replication and transcription by the elaboration of small complementary or 'antisense' RNA molecules (for a review see Weintraub, 1990; or Inouye, 1988). Evidence also now exists that eukaryotic cells elaborate antisense RNA transcripts (Kochbin and Lawrence, 1989; Krystal, Armstrong and Battey, 1990), but the physiologic role of such molecules remains controversial. Nevertheless, in 1985, Izant and Weintraub reported that a transfected expression vector could generate RNA capable of modulating eukaryotic gene expression in a target-specific manner. Actually, prior to the discovery of regulatory RNAs, several laboratories had demonstrated that synthetic oligodeoxynucleotides complementary to mRNA sequences could downregulate mRNA translation in vitro and in cells (Zamecnik and Stephenson, 1978). A profusion of reports has followed, describing the modulation of various oncogenes by both DNA and RNA antisense techniques. Such manipulations offer the possibility of combining the specificity of genetic approaches with the reversibility and temporal control of more pharmacologic approaches. The continued development of antisense technology and related delivery systems has led to initial explorations of the in-vivo utility of antisense, particularly as it relates to oligonucleotides.

However, the excitement generated by initial in-vitro successes has been tempered by the dawning realization that antisense technology is not as 'clean' as previously thought. It is both more difficult and less appealing to publish one's experimental failures, so that reports of problems and difficulties with antisense techniques have been slow to appear in the scientific literature. However, understanding the problems associated with this technology is essential for the true promise of antisense ultimately to be achieved. The purpose of this chapter is to review the anticancer applications of antisense oligonucleotides, and to describe some of the more commonly observed problems associated with their use in vitro and in vivo.

Anticancer applications of antisense oligonucleotides

The potential of antisense-directed oligonucleotides in cancer treatment has been amply demonstrated in several basic studies. Thus, Monia et al. have demonstrated specific inhibition of C-raf-1 mRNA and protein with a unique antisense sequence (Monia et al., 1996). A mismatched oligonucleotide did not generate these effects, nor did the C-raf-targeted oligonucleotide affect levels of A-raf, thus demonstrating at least a modicum of molecular specificity. These authors were also able to demonstrate dose-dependent effects of C-raf-targeted antisense on tumor xenograft growth in athymic mice, and were able to correlate these effects with loss of C-raf mRNA from tumors of treated animals. However, maximal inhibition of C-raf mRNA required continuous treatment with oligonucleotide for 13 days. Although C-raf-1 is expressed in many normal tissues and probably plays an important role in normal signal transduction processes, the authors suggest that tumors may be more sensitive to C-raf inhibition than normal tissues since prolonged exposure of mice to murine C-raf-targeted oligonucleotides gave no evidence of toxicity, although C-raf depletion could be demonstrated in multiple normal tissues.

Dean et al. have recently reported promising antitumor results in animals by targeting protein kinase C-α (Dean et al., 1996). Although protein kinase C comprises several isoforms, only the α isoform was shown to be reduced following antisense treatment, again nicely demonstrating molecular specificity. Continuous treatment of animals for two weeks with as little as 6 µg/kg per day oligonucleotide was sufficient to produce tumor growth inhibition approaching 50%, while treatment with a mismatched oligonucleotide at 6 mg/kg per day was completely ineffective (Dean et al., 1996). When animals with established tumors were treated with the protein kinase C-α-targeted oligonucleotide, clear reductions in protein kinase C-α protein level were observed in excised tumor tissue.

Cho-Chung and colleagues have recently demonstrated that antisense inhibition of protein kinase A results in tumor growth inhibition in athymic mice (Nesterova and Cho-Chung, 1995; Cho-Chung, 1996, 1997). These investigators have demonstrated that sequence-specific inhibition of the RI alpha subunit by a single injection of antisense oligonucleotide produces an inhibition of tumor growth which persists for up to two weeks. In their hands, infrequent dosing is sufficient to maintain this phenotype. Interestingly, the antisense-treated cells appear to lose their tumorigenic phenotype and begin to act more like nontransformed cells.

Future possible anticancer targets for antisense oligonucleotides are suggested by several reports wherein tumor cells transduced with antisense-producing plasmids demonstrate much reduced tumorigenic potential when injected into animals. Thus, mammary carcinoma cells expressing antisense RNA to transforming growth factor-β1 are much less tumorigenic in a syngeneic animal model (Park et al., 1997). Similarly, growth of glioblastoma cells in a syngeneic rodent model is severely compromised if the tumor cells are transduced with an antisense construct to vascular endothelial growth factor prior to their inoculation into animals (Saleh, Stacker and Wilks, 1996).

General considerations

In the application of antisense techniques to the study of cellular systems, the need for adequate controls and appropriate endpoints cannot be stressed enough. Early studies targeted reporter gene constructs such as chloramphenicol acetyl transferase and thymidine kinase to explore the specificity and utility of antisense strategies (Izant and Weintraub, 1984, 1985). These genes code for readily quantified protein products and, because they were extraneous to the cells into which they were introduced, their expression was not tied to normal cellular physiology. Interference with their expression had little impact on cell function and, as a result, interpretation of results was relatively clean and straightforward. In the case of cellular genes, the situation becomes more complex. Interference with expression can have far-reaching and unexpected results which may be difficult to distinguish from nonspecific or toxic antisense effects. Many gene products are difficult to quantitate, either because reagents do not exist or because expression is at such low levels that sensitivity becomes a problem. Investigators have occasionally been unable to document decreases in steady state target mRNA levels even though target protein levels showed dramatic declines. The reasons for this are not clear. Similarly, it has often not been possible to document antisense RNA transcripts in transfected cells even though a pronounced biologic effect is observed. Biologic endpoints as an indication of true antisense effect can be very misleading. In particular, interference with genes critical to proliferation or survival may facilitate the overgrowth of resistant, mutant or otherwise compensated populations which are not representative of the original system or its biology.

A recent editorial in the journal *Antisense Research and Development* (Stein and Krieg, 1994) has called for the use of three types of control oligonucleotides: (1) a sense control, which maintains structural features of the oligonucleotide but not base composition; (2) a scrambled control, which maintains base composition but not structural features; and (3) a mismatch control to demonstrate target hybridization specificity. As will be seen below, even these controls may not be adequate to rule out nonantisense effects of oligonucleotides.

Does oligonucleotide length affect specificity?

Among the important variables in the use of antisense oligonucleotides is certainly the length of sequence required for adequate specificity and optimal efficacy. Based on an estimate of approximately 3–4 billion base pairs in the human genome, and assuming a random distribution of bases, a number of investigators have calculated the minimum size needed to recognize a single specific sequence in the genome as between 12 and 15 bases (Woolf, Melton and Jennings, 1992). Interestingly, longer may not be better. Antisense effects in *Xenopus* oocytes have been reported with an oligonucleotide as short as 10 bases (Shuttleworth et al., 1988). Woolf et al. have pointed out that increasing an oligonucleotide beyond that minimum length would be expected to decrease, rather than increase specificity, since a longer oligonucleotide would contain more internal sequences long enough to hybridize to other mRNAs (Woolf et al., 1992). Thus, a 20-mer contains 9 different consecutive 12-mers, giving rise to approximately 11 different matches of 12 consecutive bases. Since antisense oligonucleotides as long as 21 bases are now commonly used as specific inhibitors of gene expression, the effect of mismatches on antisense efficacy becomes a very important and practical question.

In a recent study using microinjection into *Xenopus* oocytes, Woolf et al. examined the degree to which mismatched antisense phosphodiester oligonucleotides could still cause degradation of their target mRNAs via RNase H (Woolf et al., 1992). The results are disturbing. Using fibronectin as the target mRNA in *Xenopus*, the authors demonstrated that a perfectly complementary 25-mer antisense oligonucleotide produced 70% degradation of the target mRNA after six hours. However, 25-mers with 17 and 14 centrally located complementary bases caused 32% and 37% degradation, respectively. The authors demonstrated that even internal mismatches did not prevent target sequence degradation. Using another target, Vg1 mRNA, they found that a single mismatch about one-third of the way along a 13-mer antisense oligonucleotide reduced, but did not eliminate, target degradation. Thus, the fully complementary 13-mer produced 90% degradation over six hours, while the mismatch sequence caused 42% degradation over this time.

Since antisense-mediated degradation of a target sequence can be accomplished using a minimum of ten consecutive complementary bases, and non-complementary flanking sequences do not prevent antisense effects, Woolf et al. reached the conclusion that any oligonucleotide long enough to be useful as an antisense reagent would be likely to cause at least partial degradation of a large number of mRNA species. Since *Xenopus* oocytes grow at a temperature of approximately 22°C, one could hope that the more stringent hybridization conditions under which mammalian cells grow (i.e., 37°C) might eliminate this problem. However, because antisense effects have been reported in mammalian cells with sequences as small as 11 bases (Chang et al., 1991), one must at least consider the possibility of nonspecific mRNA cleavage.

Motifs within oligonucleotides can stimulate the immune system

In two reports, Yamamoto et al. (1992) and Kuramoto et al. (1992) found that certain 6-mer palindromic sequences potently induced interferon production in murine spleen cells. The most active palindromes were 5'-GACGTC-3', 5'-AGCGCT-3' and 5'-AACGTT-3'. Interferon production was accompanied by stimulation of natural killer cell activity, which could be blocked by antibodies to interferon. The authors noted that extrapalindromic sequences contributed to these effects. Thus, reducing a 45-mer oligonucleotide to a 15-mer while maintaining the 6-mer palindrome, markedly reduced stimulatory activity (Tokunaga et al., 1992). An oligonucleotide with a repeated palindrome flanked by guanylate residues demonstrated the strongest activity (Kuramoto et al., 1992). The authors also concluded that a 5'-CpG-3' motif was essential to the activity.

Interestingly, these authors initiated these studies because of earlier work demonstrating that a preparation of bacterial DNA displayed strong antitumor activity in mouse and guinea-pig (Tokunaga et al., 1984; Shimada et al., 1985). The original synthetic oligonucleotides tested were derived from sequences contained within the bacterial DNA preparation. In a more recent study, Krieg et al. (1995) reported that unmethylated CpG motifs in bacterial DNA were responsible for B cell activation, identifying this as a novel T cell-independent B cell activation pathway. Oligonucleotides with CpG-containing hexamers were also quite effective, resulting in the recruitment of more than 95% of all splenic B cells into the cell cycle. Not surprisingly, three of the four most active hexamers reported by Krieg et al. were also found to be active in the earlier studies of Yamamoto et al. (1992) and Kuramoto et al. (1992).

The importance of extrapalindromic sequence in this phenomenon is demonstrated in a study by McIntyre et al. (1993). In this study, the authors showed that a sense control oligonucleotide to NF-kB caused massive splenomegaly and B cell activation in mice. The sequence indeed contained a CpG hexamer. Although the antisense sequences also contained a CpG hexamer it was without effect, as were several other CpG-containing sequences. However, several additional unrelated CpG-containing oligonucleotides did produce B cell activation.

Krieg et al. conclude that 'it may be desirable to avoid unmethylated CpGs in antisense oligonucleotides, or at least to include controls for these effects' (Krieg et al., 1995), particularly in vivo. However, given the difficulty of designing a proper mismatched control (see above), and given the dependence of immune stimulatory effects on extrapalindromic sequences, this may prove to be a difficult task.

Oligonucleotides nonspecifically suppress [³H]thymidine incorporation

Breakdown of thymidine-containing oligonucleotides and resultant alteration of nucleotide pools can have dramatic effects on assays of cellular proliferation and DNA synthesis, such as [³H]thymidine incorporation (Matson and Krieg, 1992). This potential artifact is particularly relevant when using oligomers to study the regulation of proliferation. Because oligonucleotide degradation in serum is primarily due to 3'-exonuclease activity (Neckers et al., 1992), thymidines at or near the 3' end of an oligonucleotide are more 'inhibitory' than thymidines near the 5' end of a sequence. While apparent inhibition can be as great as 90%, this is due solely to dilution of cellular thymidine pools (with a resultant decrease in specific activity of the radioactive tracer) and not to any true growth effects.

Oligonucleotide–drug interactions

Development of oligonucleotide-based therapeutics has raised the possibility of potential combination therapy with conventional chemotherapeutic agents. It has been found that the class of anticancer drugs known collectively as DNA intercalators can bind directly to certain oligonucleotides (Stull, Zon and Szoka, 1993; Blagosklonny and Neckers, 1994). This effect was initially observed while searching for an antisense oligonucleotide to the tumor necrosis factor (TNF) receptor. As a screening assay, the ability of various sequences to block TNF-mediated in-vitro cytoxicity was being assessed. This assay relies on small concentrations of actinomycin D to potentiate effects of TNF. Surprisingly, many different oligonucleotides, related and unrelated to the TNF receptor mRNA sequence, reversed TNF toxicity. Upon closer examination, the effect could not be attributed to TNF receptor downregulation, but to interference with the activity of actinomycin D. Indeed, using a fluorescent derivative of actinomycin D, it was possible to demonstrate direct binding of oligonucleotide to drug. Binding affinity was dependent on oligonucleotide length and guanosine content, but was not sequence dependent (Blagosklonny and Neckers, 1994).

The cytoprotective effect of all oligonucleotides was completely dependent on their ability to bind actinomycin. More importantly, these oligonucleotides were also able to abrogate the cytotoxicity of other DNA intercalators, including adriamycin and daunomycin. The toxicity of other DNA-damaging agents, including mitomycin C, cisplatin, VP-16, and camptothecin, was not affected (Blagosklonny and Neckers, 1994). The mechanism by which single-stranded oligonucleotides bind to DNA intercalators appears to involve stacked complexes of drug and DNA (Wadkins and Jovin, 1991).

Phosphorothioate oligonucleotides directly interact with proteins

A major hurdle in the development of antisense oligonucleotides has been the stability of the molecules themselves in serum-containing media and in cells. Unmodified phosphodiester (Po) oligonucleotides are very susceptible to degradation by cellular nucleases. Po oligonucleotides microinjected into a *Xenopus* embryo have half-lives of less than 30 minutes (see Neckers et al. (1992) for review). Similar in-vivo results were obtained when Po oligonucleotides were injected directly into the brains of rodents (Whitesell et al., 1993; Ogawa et al., 1995). Studies of fluorescent oligonucleotides administered in vitro to mammalian cells have demonstrated degradation of Po compounds within three hours (Akhtar, Kole and Juliano, 1991; Iverson et al., 1992). In contrast, phosphorothioate (Ps) oligonucleotides are highly resistant to nuclease degradation (Campbell, Bacon and Wickstrom, 1990; for review see Neckers et al., 1992). Because this modification is relatively easy to make and is chemically stable, it has become the modification of choice for production of antisense oligonucleotides stable enough for in-vitro and in-vivo use.

Evidence has been accumulating, however, that incorporation of phosphorothioate moieties into oligonucleotides makes these molecules much 'stickier' than unmodified oligonucleotides, particularly with respect to direct protein binding. An early study by Cazenave et al. (1989) tested antisense phosphorothioates in both a frog oocyte system and a wheat-germ extract in-vitro translation system, and demonstrated that, while phosphorothioates were effective antisense molecules in-vitro and in vivo at submicromolar concentrations, at 1–10 micromolar concentrations these oligonucleotides could nonspecifically inhibit protein synthesis. The authors concluded that nonspecific inhibition of protein synthesis was occurring because the Ps oligonucleotides were binding to enzymes involved in protein synthesis.

Ps oligonucleotides are strong sulfated polyanions. Naturally occurring polyanions bind and sequester various growth factors to basement membranes. Synthetic sulfated polyanions, such as suramin, heparin, dextran, and pentosan polysulfate, can mimic naturally occurring polyanions by themselves, binding to a variety of growth factors, including members of the fibroblast growth factor family (FGFs), platelet-derived growth factor (PDGF), and vascular endothelial growth factor (Wellstein et al., 1991; Zugmaier, Lippman and Wellstein, 1993). These polyanions block the binding of growth factors to their cell surface receptors. Like them, Ps oligonucleotides also antagonize the binding of both FGF and PDGF to receptors on the surface of 3T3 fibroblasts and other cells (Stein and Krieg, 1994). Ps oligonucleotides, like heparin, also release growth factors already bound to extracellular matrix (Stein and Krieg, 1994).

Other proteins which interact with and are inhibited by both Ps oligonucleotides and other sulfated polyanions include recombinant soluble CD4, HIV-1 reverse transcriptase, HIV gp120, RNase H, DNA polymerase alpha and beta, and protein kinase C (Gao et al., 1992; Maury et al., 1992; Stein et al., 1993a, 1993b; Yakubov et al., 1993). The interaction of Ps oligonucleotides with these proteins is somewhat length dependent but seems not to depend on sequence. In all cases, when a similar effect is observed with unmodified phosphodiester oligonucleotides, it is much weaker and/or requires 10–100 times more oligonucleotide.

Ps oligonucleotide inhibition of protein kinase C and RNase H is problematic for antisense experiments. Stein et al. (1993b) have found that SdC28, a Ps homopolymer of cytidine (28-mer), is able directly to inhibit the beta 1 isoform of protein kinase C with an IC_{50} of 1 μM. Other protein kinase C inhibitors appear to antagonize the cellular uptake of oligonucleotides, raising the possibility that, at low micromolar concentrations, Ps oligonucleotides will block their own cellular uptake.

At the same time, Gao et al. (1992) have reported that SdC28 can inhibit RNase H, the enzyme thought to be primarily involved in mediating antisense activity. Using sequence-specific antisense Ps oligonucleotides, these authors found that, in the presence of the complementary mRNA, they could observe a biphasic effect dependent on oligonucleotide concentration. At oligonucleotide concentrations less than or equal to the concentration of the target mRNA,

RNA cleavage could be demonstrated, suggesting RNase H activity. However, when Ps oligonucleotide concentration rose above the concentration of the target, RNA cleavage became progressively less, suggesting inhibition of RHase H activity by excess Ps oligonucleotide. Since it is impossible precisely to titrate antisense oligonucleotide concentration in cells or in vivo, the possibility distinctly exists that a Ps antisense oligonucleotide would be likely to inhibit activity of the very enzyme responsible for mediating antisense effects.

Ps oligonucleotides also activate the nuclear transcription factor Sp1 in a sequence-independent and length-independent manner (Perez et al., 1994). This effect is similar to that observed following treatment with the sulfated polyanion suramin. Induction occurs in both transformed and untransformed cells of both murine and human origin. Since Sp1 participates in transcriptional regulation of many diverse cellular promoters, nonspecific induction of this transcription factor by Ps oligonucleotides could lead to unexpected biological responses, whether or not specific antisense effects could be observed.

Sequence-specific protein recognition by phosphorothioate and unmodified oligonucleotides

Ps oligonucleotides cannot be as efficiently end-labeled with T4 polynucleotide kinase as can unmodified oligonucleotides. Teasdale et al. have recently reported that this is partly due to direct inhibition of the kinase by phosphorothioates (Teasdale et al., 1994). Inhibition was dependent on both the length of the oligonucleotide (the longer the more inhibitory) and the number of Ps linkages in the molecule. Intriguingly, some sequence specificity to the inhibition was also noted. For example, a 12-base homopolymer of cytidine was 100 times more inhibitory than a 12-base heteropolymer. The inhibitory activity of several heteropolymers of identical length was also found to vary over 1000-fold. Potential sequence motifs responsible for inhibition remain to be identified.

Direct oligonucleotide inhibition of the oncogenic tyrosine kinase, p210[bcr-abl] has recently been reported by Bergan et al. (1994, 1995). While screening for an antisense oligonucleotide, the authors found instead a sequence which directly inhibited the enzymatic activity of the kinase in vitro and in vivo without affecting its protein level. Inhibition was length and sequence dependent, requiring at least one GGC motif in a 21-base molecule. Interestingly, while a Ps oligonucleotide of appropriate sequence was inhibitory, an unmodified version of the same sequence was even more inhibitory, with an IC_{50} of less than 1 μM. However, the same sequence (non-Ps) containing a 2'-methoxy modification of the sugar moiety was completely ineffective as a kinase inhibitor. Thus, negative charge alone, in the context of sequence, is not sufficient to achieve inhibition.

The kinase specificity of this oligonucleotide was demonstrated by the fact that several other tyrosine and serine/threonine kinases required at least one log more oligonucleotide before inhibition could be observed. Inhibition was noncompetitive with respect to ATP, but could be antagonized by addition of a substrate protein, suggesting that the oligonucleotide bound to a substrate recognition site on the p210 protein.

Perhaps the finding of this study most relevant to antisense technology is that this direct protein-binding effect is dependent on both sequence and secondary structure of the oligonucleotide. Changing the character of the phosphate linkage or the sugar moiety without changing the sequence would not be expected to affect hybridization to target mRNA, but these alterations had profound effects on oligonucleotide inhibition of kinase activity.

Perhaps the most carefully controlled example of a physiologically significant direct oligonucleotide/protein interaction is a report by Bock et al. (1992), describing identification of a consensus 15-base sequence capable of inhibiting thrombin activity. This sequence was identified by screening a random library containing approximately 10^{13} oligonucleotides. The consensus sequence, at 100 nM concentration, was able to increase clotting time nearly seven-fold, while a scrambled sequence was without effect. Thus, as in the example of p210[bcr-abl], although thrombin has at least two anion-binding sites, electrostatic interactions cannot be solely responsible for the inhibitory effects observed.

Phosphorothioate oligonucleotides can inhibit adhesion

Several groups have demonstrated an inhibitory effect of Ps oligonucleotides on cellular adhesion (Watson, Pon and Shiu, 1992; Yaswen et al., 1993; Chavany, Connell and Neckers, 1995; Maltese et al., 1995). Watson, Pon and Shiu (1992) first reported that a Ps oligonucleotide targeting the c-*myc* oncogene inhibited the adhesion of MCF7 breast cancer cells. This effect appeared to be sequence specific, since the sense oligonucleotide and another irrelevant antisense oligonucleotide were without effect. However, the effect was not mediated via an antisense mechanism, since the authors could not demonstrate any alteration in either c-myc mRNA or protein.

More recently, Yaswen et al. (1993) reported similar findings with a Ps c-*myc* antisense oligonucleotide and other Ps sequences. These authors extended the work of Watson, Pon and Shiu by making the observation that all oligonucleotides which inhibited adhesion had in common a so-called dG quartet – that is, a motif of four contiguous guanosine residues – embedded in the overall sequence. They suggested that Ps oligonucleotides containing a dG quartet could somehow be inhibitory to cellular adhesion through undefined nonantisense mechanisms.

However, Maltese et al. (1995) have found that sequences surrounding the dG quartet motif also contribute to an oligonucleotide's antiadhesive properties, making the dG quartet essential but not sufficient for adhesion inhibition. Recent results of Chavany et al. (1995) complicate the situation even further. These investigators found that both sequence and phosphorothioate content contribute to antiadhesion phenomena. Working with the same c-*myc* antisense oligonucleotide as Watson, Pon and Shiu, and Yaswen et al., they observed no sequence specificity to the antiadhesion effect if Ps oligonucleotides were used. As one might expect, oligonucleotides containing a dG quartet were more inhibitory to adhesion than were oligonucleotides lacking this motif. However, several oligonucleotides which did or did not contain a dG motif were equally inhibitory on cell growth in a sequence-nonspecific fashion.

In contrast, when the phosphorothioate content of these oligonucleotides was reduced to 53% (by capping the oligonucleotide on either end with phosphorothioate linkages but leaving the remainder of the molecule unmodified), a sequence-specific antiadhesive effect became apparent. The c-myc antisense sequence was strongly antiadhesive, but none of the control sequences was adhesive. Controls included dG quartet-containing oligonucleotides, including a 2-base mismatched antisense oligonucleotide. Thus, in these experiments, completely phosphorothioating the oligonucleotides masked a c-*myc* antisense sequence-specific antiadhesive effect for which a dG quartet alone was not sufficient.

These results are in keeping with the findings of Brown et al. (1994), who recently reported strong and rather promiscuous intracellular protein binding by Ps oligonucleotides. These authors found that sequence-independent protein binding of Ps oligonucleotides was directly proportional to the degree of Ps content of the oligonucleotides. As in the study of Chavany et al., the authors found that reducing the Ps content of an oligonucleotide was sufficient to restore its sequence-specific protein interactions (i.e., sequence-specific double-stranded oligonucleotide interactions with transcription factors).

However, the antiadhesive properties of the c-*myc* antisense oligonucleotide reported by Chavany et al. are not mediated via antisense effects on c-*myc* because: (1) washing pretreated cells free of extracellular oligonucleotide completely abolished the effect without reversing the inhibition of c-*myc* protein; and (2) addition of treated cells to fibronectin-coated culture dishes also abolished the effect without interfering in the inhibition of c-myc protein. Also, neither unmodified phosphodiester oligonucleotides nor phosphoramidate-modified oligonucleotides were found to be antiadhesive, although antisense effects toward c-myc could still be demonstrated.

Do suitable controls exist for antisense experiments?

Given these examples of sequence-specific and nonspecific nonantisense effects of oligonucleotides, one must readdress the question of controls. At the beginning of this chapter are listed several proposals for appropriate controls made by the editors of the journal *Antisense Research and Development*. These include a sense control, a scrambled control, and a mismatch control.

The previous discussion has pointed out that sense and scrambled controls may not contain biologically active motifs found in the antisense sequence. At the same time, mismatch oligonucleotides, depending on overall length, may not control for hybridization specificity. In addition, the relative position of mismatches within an oligonucleotide sequence is critical to loss of activity (Woolf et al., 1992; Maltese et al., 1995). While a single mismatch nucleotide can in some cases abolish antisense activity, in many cases even several mismatches fail to abrogate activity (Maltese et al., 1995). The success or failure of mismatches in abrogating antisense activity is completely contextual, and no rules can be codified as to the proper method of choosing which bases to mismatch. Indeed, it is our opinion that each and every oligonucleotide be considered a unique drug, for which no ideal control exists. Thus, even those antisense experiments which apply the most stringent conditions to validate activity cannot unequivocally demonstrate that antisense is the sole mechanism mediating a given biological phenomenon.

Can the nonantisense effects of oligonucleotides be of clinical utility?

Even though the nonantisense effects of particular oligonucleotides may be problematic under certain circumstances, at least some of these effects may prove to be of clinical utility.

Earlier in this chapter, an aptameric inhibitor of the protein tyrosine kinase is described that is characteristically expressed in chronic myelogenous leukemia (CML) cells, $p210^{bcr-abl}$ (Bergan et al., 1994, 1995). This inhibitor is capable of reducing the cellular phosphotyrosine content and clonagenicity when administered to CML cells in vitro, and a similar activity has recently been demonstrated when given in vivo (R. Bergan et al., unpublished observations). However, the oligonucleotide does not affect normal marrow progenitors, and thus allows for the ex-vivo purging of CML-containing marrow. In a preclinical murine model, such treatment resulted in complete elimination of tumor in 80% of immunocompromised animals reconstituted with oligonucleotide-treated marrow (R. Bergan et al., unpublished observations).

CpG motifs in oligonucleotides trigger the activation of B, T, and natural killer cells, partly but not entirely by stimulating coordinate secretion of interleukin-6, interleukin-12 and interferon gamma (Kuramoto et al., 1992; Yamamoto et al., 1992; Krieg et al., 1995; Klinman et al., 1996; Yi et al., 1996). Such stimulation is very potent, even at oligonucleotide concentrations of 1 μM. Immune-stimulating, CpG-containing oligonucleotides may prove clinically useful anticancer agents as adjuvants and biological response modifiers.

Another clinical application of an aptameric oligonucleotide is in the area of anticoagulation. Recently, a novel 15-mer has been described which is able to bind to and rapidly inactivate thrombin (Bock et al., 1992). Upon infusion of this aptamer in monkeys, maximal anticoagulation was achieved within ten minutes. Within ten minutes of infusion termination, coagulation parameters returned to normal (Griffin et al., 1993). The rapid onset of action and short in-vivo half-life of this aptamer may have distinct advantages in certain clinical settings.

Interestingly, the thrombin aptamer forms a quadruplex structure in solution, consisting of two G-quartets connected by two TT loops and one TGT loop (Macaya et al., 1993). Another aptameric oligonucleotide, with affinity to the cationic V3 loop of the envelope glycoprotein gp120 of HIV, has also been described to form a quadruplex in solution (Wyatt et al., 1994). The antiviral activity of this compound (TTGGGGTT) is due to its ability to inhibit HIV envelope-mediated cell fusion and virus binding to cells, for which the quadruplex structure appears necessary (Buckheit et al., 1994). This oligonucleotide is a potential candidate for use in anti-HIV chemotherapy.

Conclusion

The results demonstrate that, although antisense inhibition in the absence of other activities may be difficult, if not impossible, to achieve, this may still prove to be a fruitful approach for anticancer therapy. In addition, one should not ignore the ability of certain novel backbone-containing oligonucleotides to interact with proteins as well as RNA (and DNA). Chemically modified oligonucleotides represent a unique class of combinatorial drug whose true potential has yet to be fully realized.

References

Akhtar, S., Kole, R. and Juliano, R. L. (1991). Stability of antisense DNA oligodeoxynucleotide analogs in cellular extracts and sera. *Life Sciences*, **49**: 1793.

Bergan, R., Connell, Y., Fahmy, B., Kyle, E. and Neckers, L. (1994). Aptameric inhibition of p210[bcr-abl] tyrosine kinase autophosphorylation by oligodeoxynucleotides of defined sequence and backbone structure. *Nucleic Acids Research*, **22**: 2150.

Bergan, R. C., Kyle, E., Connell, Y. and Neckers, L. (1995). Inhibition of protein tyrosine kinase activity in intact cells by the aptameric action of oligodeoxynucleotides. *Antisense Research and Development*, **5**: 33.

Blagosklonny, M. V. and Neckers, L. M. (1994). Oligonucleotides protect cells from the cytotoxicity of several anti-cancer chemotherapeutic drugs. *Anti-Cancer Drugs*, **5**: 437.

Bock, L. C., Griffin, L. C., Latham, J. A., Vermass, E. H. and Toole, J. J. (1992). Selection of single-stranded DNA molecules that bind and inhibit human thrombin. *Nature*, **355**: 564.

Brown, D. A., Kang, S.-H., Gryaznov, S. M., DeDionisio, L., Heidenreich, O., Sullivan, S., Xu, X. and Nerenberg, M. I. (1994). Effect of phosphorothioate modification of oligodeoxynucleotides on specific protein binding. *Journal of Biological Chemistry*, **269**: 26801.

Buckheit, R. W., Roberson, J. L., Lackman-Smith, C., Wyatt, J. R., Vickers, T. A. and Ecker, D. J. (1994). Potent and specific inhibition of HIV envelope-mediated cell fusion and virus binding by G quartet-forming oligonucleotide (ISIS 5320). *Antisense Research and Development*, **10**: 1497.

Campbell, J. M., Bacon, T. A. and Wickstrom, E. (1990). Oligodeoxynucleotide phosphorothioate stability in subcellular extracts, culture media, serum and cerebrospinal fluid. *Journal of Biochemical and Biophysical Methods*, **20**: 259.

Cazenave, C., Stein, C. A., Loreau, N., Thuong, N. T., Neckers, L. M., Subasinghe, C., Helene, C., Cohen, J. S. and Toulme, J.-J. (1989). Comparative inhibition of rabbit globin mRNA translation by modified antisense oligodeoxynucleotides. *Nucleic Acids Research*, **17**: 4255.

Chang, E. H., Miller, P. S., Cushman, C., Devadas, K., Pirollo, K. F., Ts'o, P. O. P. and Yu, Z. P. (1991). Antisense inhibition of ras p21 expression that is sensitive to a point mutation. *Biochemistry*, **30**: 8283.

Chavany, C., Connell, Y. and Neckers, L. (1995). Contribution of sequence and phosphorothioate content to inhibition of cell growth and adhesion caused by c-myc antisense oligomers. *Molecular Pharmacology*, **48**: 738.

Cho-Chung, Y. S. (1996). Protein-kinase A-directed antisense restrains cancer growth: sequence-specific inhibition of gene expression. *Antisense Nucleic Acid Drug Developments*, **6**: 237.

Cho-Chung, Y. S. (1997). Antisense DNA toward type 1 protein kinase A produces sustained inhibition of tumor growth. *Proceedings of the Association of American Physicians*, **109**: 23.

Dean, N., McKay, R., Miraglia, L., Howard, R., Cooper, S., Giddings, J., Nicklin, P., Meister, L., Ziel, R., Geiger, T., Muller, M. and Fabbro, D. (1996). Inhibition of growth of human tumor cell lines in nude mice by an antisense oligonucleotide inhibitor of protein kinase C-α expression. *Cancer Research*, **56**: 3499.

Gao, W.-Y., Han, F.-S., Storm, C., Egan, W. and Cheng, Y.-C. (1992). Phosphorothioate oligonucleotides are inhibitors of human DNA polymerases and RNase H: Implications for antisense technology. *Molecular Pharmacology*, **41**: 223.

Griffin, L. C., Tidmarsh, G. F., Bock, L. C., Toole, J. J. and Leung, L. L. (1993). In vivo anticoagulant properties of a novel nucleotide-based thrombin inhibitor and demonstration of regional anticoagulation in extra corporeal circuits. *Blood*, **81**: 3271.

Inouye, M. (1988). Antisense RNA: its functions and applications in gene regulation – a review. *Gene*, **72**: 25.

Iverson, P. L., Zhu, S., Meyer, A. and Zon, G. (1992). Cellular uptake and subcellular distribution of phosphorothioate oligonucleotides into cultured cells. *Antisense Research and Development*, **2**: 211.

Izant, J. G. and Weintraub, H. (1984). Inhibition of thymidine kinase gene expression by antisense RNA: a molecular approach to genetic analyses. *Cell*, **36**: 1007.

Izant, J. G. and Weintraub, H. (1985). Constitutive and conditional suppression of exogenous and endogenous genes by anti-sense RNA. *Science*, **229**: 345.

Klinman, D. M., Yi, A. K., Beaucage, S. L., Conover, J. and Krieg, A. M. (1996). CpG motifs present in bacterial DNA rapidly induce lymphocytes to secrete interleukin-6, interleukin-12, and interferon gamma. *Proceedings of the National Academy of Sciences of the United States of America*, **93**: 2879.

Kochbin, S. and Lawrence, J. J. (1989). An antisense RNA involved in p53 mRNA maturation in murine erythroleukemia cells induced to differentiate. *EMBO Journal*, **8**: 4107.

Krieg, A. M., Yi, A.-K., Matson, S., Waldschmidt, T. J., Bishop, G. A., Teasdale, R., Koretsky, G. A. and Klinman, D. M. (1995). CpG motifs in bacterial DNA trigger direct B-cell activation. *Nature*, **374**: 546.

Krystal, G. W., Armstrong, B. C. and Battey, J. F. (1990). N-myc mRNA forms an RNA–RNA duplex with endogenous antisense transcripts. *Molecular and Cellular Biology*, **10**: 4180.

Kuramoto, E., Yano, O., Kimura, Y., Baba, M., Maino, T., Yamamoto, S., Yamamoto, T., Kataoka, T. and Tokunaga, T. (1992). Oligonucleotide sequences required for natural killer cell activation. *Japanese Journal of Cancer Research*, **83**: 1128.

Macaya, R. F., Schultze, P., Smith, F. W., Roe, J. A. and Feigon, J. (1993). Thrombin-binding DNA aptamer forms a unimolecular quadruplex structure in solution. *Proceedings of the National Academy of Sciences of the United States of America*, **90**: 3745.

Maltese, J.-Y., Sharma, H. W., Vassilev, L. and Narayanan, R. (1995). Sequence context of antisense RelA/NF-kB phosphorothioates determines specificity. *Nucleic Acids Research*, **23**: 1146.

Matson, S. and Krieg, A. M. (1992). Nonspecific suppression of [^{3}H]thymidine incorporation by 'control' oligonucleotides. *Antisense Research and Development*, **2**: 325.

Maury, G., Alaoui, A. E., Morvan, F., Muller, B., Imbach, J.-L. and Goody, R. S. (1992). Template-phosphorothioate oligonucleotide duplexes as inhibitors of HIV-1 reverse transcriptase. *Biochemical and Biophysical Research Communications*, **186**: 1249.

McIntyre, K. W., Lombard-Gillooly, K., Perez, J. R., Kunsch, C., Sarmiento, U. M., Larigan, J. D., Landreth, K. T. and Narayanan, R. (1993). A sense phosphorothioate oligonucleotide directed to the initiation codon of transcription factor NF-kB p65 causes sequence-specific immune stimulation. *Antisense Research and Development*, **3**: 309.

Monia, B. P., Johnston, J. F., Geiger, T., Muller, M. and Fabbro, D. (1996). Antitumor activity of a phosphorothioate antisense oligodeoxynucleotide targeted against C-*raf* kinase. *Nature Medicine*, **2**: 668.

Neckers, L., Whitesell, L., Rosolen, A. and Geselowitz, D. (1992). Antisense inhibition of gene expression. *Critical Reviews in Oncogenesis*, **3**: 175.
Nesterova, M. and Cho-Chung, Y. S. (1995). A single-injection protein kinase A-directed antisense treatment to inhibit tumour growth. *Nature Medicine*, **1**: 528.
Ogawa, S., Brown, H. E., Okano, H. J. and Pfaff, D. W. (1995). Cellular uptake of intracerebrally administered oligodeoxynucleotides in mouse brain. *Regulatory Peptides*, **59**: 143.
Park, J. A., Wang, E., Kurt, R. A., Schluter, S. F., Hersch, E. M. and Akporiaye, E. T. (1997). Expression of an antisense transforming growth factor-β1 transgene reduces tumorigenicity of EMT6 mammary tumor cells. *Cancer Gene Therapy*, **4**: 42.
Perez, J. R., Li, Y., Stein, C. A., Majumder, S., Oorschot, A. V. and Narayanan, R. (1994). Sequence-independent induction of Sp1 transcription factor activity by phosphorothioate oligodeoxynucleotides. *Proceedings of the National Academy of Sciences of the United States of America*, **91**: 5957.
Saleh, M., Stacker, S. A. and Wilks, A. F. (1996). Inhibition of growth of C6 glioma cells in vivo by expression of antisense vascular endothelial growth factor sequence. *Cancer Research*, **56**: 393.
Shimada, S., Yano, O., Inoue, H., Kuramoto, E., Fukuda, T., Yamamoto, H., Kataoka, T. and Tokunaga, T. (1985). Antitumor activity of the DNA fraction from *Mycobacterium bovis* BCG. II. Effects on various syngeneic mouse tumors. *Journal of the National Cancer Institute*, **74**: 681.
Shuttleworth, J., Matthews, G., Dale, L., Baker, C. and Colman, A. (1988). Antisense oligodeoxyribonucleotide-directed cleavage of maternal mRNA in *Xenopus* oocytes and embryos. *Gene*, **72**: 267.
Stein, C. A., Cleary, A., Yakubov, L. and Lederman, S. (1993a). Phosphorothioate oligodeoxynucleotides bind to the third variable loop domain (V3) of HIV-1 gp120. *Antisense Research and Development*, **3**: 19.
Stein, C. A., Tonkinson, J. L., Zhang, L.-M., Yakubov, L., Gervasoni, J., Taub, R. and Rotenberg, S. A. (1993b). Dynamics of the internalization of phosphodiester oligodeoxynucleotides in HL60 cells. *Biochemistry*, **32**: 4855.
Stein, C. A. and Krieg, A. M. (1994). Problems in interpretation of data derived from in vitro and in vivo use of antisense oligodeoxynucleotides. *Antisense Research and Development*, **4**: 67.
Stull, R. A., Zon, G. and Szoka, F. C. (1993). Single-stranded phosphodiester and phosphorothioate oligonucleotides bind actinomycin D and interfere with tumor necrosis factor-induced lysis in the L929 cytotoxicity assay. *Antisense Research and Development*, **3**: 295.
Teasadle, R. M., Matson, S. J., Fisher, E. and Krieg, A. M. (1994). Inhibition of T4 polynucleotide kinase activity by phosphorothioate and chimeric oligodeoxynucleotides. *Antisense Research and Development*, **4**: 295.
Tokunaga, T., Yamamoto, H., Shimada, S., Abe, H., Fukuda, T., Fujisawa, Y., Furutani, Y., Yano, O., Kataoka, T., Sudo, T., Makiguchi, N. and Suganuma, T. (1984). Antitumor activity of deoxyribonucleic acid fraction from *Mycobacterium bovis* GCG. I. Isolation, physicochemical characterization, and antitumor activity. *Journal of the National Cancer Institute*, **72**: 955.
Tokunaga, T., Yano, O., Kuramoto, E., Kimura, Y., Yamamoto, T., Kataoka, T. and Yamamoto, S. (1992). Synthetic oligonucleotides with particular base sequences from the cDNA encoding proteins of *Mycobacterium bovis* BCG induce interferons and activate natural killer cells. *Microbiological Immunology*, **36**: 55.

Wadkins, R. M. and Jovin, T. M. (1991). Actinomycin D and 7-aminoactinomycin D binding to single-stranded DNA. *Biochemistry*, **30**: 9469.
Watson, P. H., Pon, R. T. and Shiu, R. P. C. (1992). Inhibition of cell adhesion to plastic substratum by phosphorothioate oligonucleotide. *Experimental Cell Research*, **202**: 391.
Weintraub, H. M. (1990). Antisense RNA and DNA. *Scientific American*, **262**: 40.
Wellstein, A., Zugmaier, G., Califano, J., Kern, F., Paik, S. and Lippman, M. (1991). Tumor growth dependent on Kaposi's sarcoma-derived fibroblast growth factor inhibited by pentosan polysulfate. *Journal of the National Cancer Institute*, **83**: 716.
Whitesell, L., Geselowitz, D., Chavany, C., Fahmy, B., Walbridge, S., Alger, J. R. and Neckers, L. M. (1993). Stability, clearance and disposition of intraventricularly administered oligodeoxynucleotides – implications for therapeutic application within the central nervous system. *Proceedings of the National Academy of Sciences of the United States of America*, **90**: 4665.
Woolf, T. M., Melton, D. A. and Jennings, C. G. B. (1992). Specificity of antisense oligonucleotides in vivo. *Proceedings of the National Academy of Sciences of the United States of America*, **89**: 7305.
Wyatt, J. R., Vickers, T. A., Roberson, J. L., Buckheit, R. W., Klimkait, T., DeBaets, E., Davis, P. W., Rayner, B., Imbach, J. L. and Ecker, D. (1994). G-quartet structure is a potent inhibitor of HIV envelope-mediated cell fusion. *Proceedings of the National Academy of Sciences of the United States of America*, **91**: 1356.
Yakubov, L., Khaled, Z., Zhang, L.-M., Truneh, A., Vlassov, V. and Stein, C. A. (1993). Mode of interaction of oligodeoxynucleotides with recombinant sCD4. *Journal of Biological Chemistry*, **268**: 18818.
Yamamoto, S., Yamamoto, T., Kataoka, T., Kuramoto, E., Yano, O. and Tokunaga, T. (1992). Unique palindromic sequences in synthetic oligonucleotides are required to induce INF and augment INF-mediated natural killer activity. *Journal of Immunology*, **148**: 4072.
Yaswen, P., Stampfer, M. R., Ghosh, K. and Cohen, J. S. (1993). Effects of sequence of thioated oligonucleotides on cultured human mammary epithelial cells. *Antisense Research and Development*, **3**: 67.
Yi, A. K., Chace, J. H., Cowdery, J. S. and Krieg, A. M. (1996). Interferon-gamma promotes IL-6 and IgM secretion in response to CpG motifs in bacterial DNA and oligodeoxynucleotides. *Journal of Immunology*, **156**: 558.
Zamecnik, P. C. and Stephenson, M. L. (1978). Inhibition of Rous sarcoma virus replication and cell transformation by a specific oligodeoxynucleotide. *Proceedings of the National Academy of Sciences of the United States of America*, **75**: 280.
Zugmaier, G., Lippman, M. and Wellstein, A. (1993). Inhibition by pentosan polysulfate (PPS) of heparin-binding growth factors released from tumor cells and blockage by PPS of tumor cell growth in animals. *Journal of the National Cancer Institute*, **84**: 1716.

9

Current status of gene marking and gene therapy in oncology clinical trials

CYNTHIA A. RICHARDS

After much public, scientific, and regulatory debate, the first clinical trial involving gene marking was initiated on May 22, 1989. Less than seven years later, over 600 patients had been enrolled in clinical gene transfer/gene therapy protocols at numerous institutions around the world. About 70% of these trials have studied oncology patients, but trials treating inborn genetic disorders such as adenosine deaminase deficiency, cystic fibrosis, and famial hypercholesterolemia, and acquired diseases such as AIDS, are also under way (Table 9.1; for review see Miller, 1992; Morgan and Anderson, 1993; Crystal, 1995). The lack of any unexpected or untoward problems in the early trials has led to a profusion of gene marking/gene therapy protocols. In addition, the trend over time has been a shift from ex-vivo gene marking toward in-vivo gene therapy protocols. New protocols are now being approved more quickly by the appropriate regulatory agencies as the public, scientific, and regulatory communities have become more comfortable with this emerging technology. In fact the need for any special regulatory overview of gene therapy protocols is currently under review (Marshall, 1995).

Current clinical gene marker/gene therapy protocols in oncology can be divided into four broad groups based on the target cell population – that is, the type of cells being genetically modified (Table 9.2). The first group of protocols involves the genetic modification of tumor-infiltrating lymphocytes (TIL). Initial marking studies are addressing questions about TIL trafficking and the general safety of gene marking/gene therapy protocols. The second group of protocols covers the genetic modification of bone marrow stem cells before autologous bone marrow transplant (ABMT). These trials are addressing fundamental questions about ABMT. For instance, does autologous marrow harvested during clinical remission contain tumor cells that contribute to disease relapse, and does the transplanted marrow contribute to hematopoietic reconstitution? The third broad group of protocols is studying genetically

166

Table 9.1. *Gene-marker and gene-therapy*
protocols in the USA and Europe*

Characterized by disease
31 Gene-marking trials
  28 in oncology
  3 other
135 Gene-therapy trials
  88 in oncology
  12 for HIV
  16 for cystic fibrosis
  3 for Gaucher disease
  16 for various monogenic and vascular diseases
Characterized by gene delivery site and vehicle
101 ex-vivo gene delivery
  90 retrovirus
  9 cationic liposome
  2 other
65 in-vivo gene delivery
  19 retrovirus
  14 cationic liposome
  21 adenovirus
  11 other

---

*As of September 1995, information from 125
Recombinant DNA Advisory Committee-approved
US protocols and 41 European protocols.

modified allogeneic tumor vaccines. The fourth, and most diverse, group of trials involves the genetic modification of autologous tumor cells. Several trials in this group involve the ex-vivo modification of cultured autologous cells. However, in most of the trials in this group gene transfer is attempted directly to the tumor in situ. Numerous investigators are trying to enhance the immune system's ability to recognize and eradicate tumor cells. Others are studying the safety and feasibility of delivering suicide, antisense, or tumor suppresser genes to tumors in situ.

Genetic modification of tumor-infiltrating lymphocytes

Tumor-infiltrating lymphocytes are lymphoid cells with unique lytic specificity for autologous tumor that traffic to and infiltrate solid tumors. There are currently six clinical trials involving gene transfer into, or gene therapy using, TIL. Five of the trials are gene marker studies that address important questions about the in-vivo distribution and survival of TIL. The sixth trial

Table 9.2. *Gene-marker and gene-therapy clinical trials in oncology**

Target cells	Marker	Therapy	Delivery method			Site of gene delivery	
			Retrovirus	Other virus	Nonviral	Ex vivo	In vivo
TIL†	6	3	8	0	1	9	0
Bone marrow, PBSC	20	7	27	0	0	27	0
Allogeneic cells	0	9	7	0	2	9	0
Autologous tumor‡	2	69	37	22	12	30	41
Totals	28	88	79	22	15	75	41

*USA and Europe as of September 1995.
†Also includes cytotoxic T lymphocytes.
‡Includes five protocols with gene-modified fibroblasts and two muscle vaccinations.
PBSC, peripheral blood stem cells.

includes studies directed towards the same distribution and survival questions as well as assessment of the safety and efficacy of tumor necrosis factor (TNF)-modified TIL. In addition to addressing basic questions about TIL biology, these trials are helping to answer fundamental questions about the safety and efficacy of retroviral-mediated gene transfer. All six trials use replication-defective retroviral vectors to transduce ex-vivo cultured, autologous TIL.

The first human gene marker trial was initiated by S. Rosenberg and his collaborators at the National Cancer Institute (NCI), Bethesda, Maryland, on May 22, 1989 (Rosenberg et al., 1990b). The trial was essentially a straightforward, minor amendment to an existing clinical protocol that was examining the effect of TIL and interleukin-2 (IL-2) in patients with advanced metastatic melanoma. The adoptive transfer of TIL and interleukin-2 (IL-2) has been shown to mediate tumor regression in some patients with advanced malignant melanoma (Rosenberg et al., 1988). The purpose of the amendment was to provide a means, not previously available, to study the survival and in-vivo distribution of reinfused autologous TIL. Investigators predicted that the knowledge gained from these experiments would enable the optimization of TIL therapies and an evaluation of the safety and feasibility of augmenting TIL immunotherapy by introducing therapeutic genes into TIL.

Prior to gene marking technology, nuclear medicine scans and sequential tumor biopsies had indicated that TIL radiolabeled with indium-111 localized to tumor deposits (Fisher et al., 1989). However, several factors including the 2.8-day half-life of indium-111, the tendency of TIL spontaneously to release indium-111, and the damage caused by the autoirradiation of the labeled TIL, limited the trafficking studies and prevented the collection of any data on long-term in-vivo distribution and survival. The techniques of efficient retroviral-mediated gene transfer and the polymerase chain reaction (PCR) combined with the availability of dominant selectable marker genes, such as neomycin phosphotransferase, which confers resistance to the neomycin analog G418, made it possible to contemplate long-term in-vivo distribution and survival studies of reinfused genetically marked TIL.

There are a number of advantages to genetically marking cells with the neomycin-resistance gene (*neo*^R) via a retroviral vector. First, retroviral vectors efficiently integrate into the cell's chromosomes where they are permanently maintained and subsequently passed on without dilution, reutilization, or sequestration, to all progeny as long as the cells survive. Also, marking cells with retroviral vectors is a simple technical procedure that does not expose the marked cells to toxic compounds or radiation, which might alter the function of the marked cell. And finally, the *neo*^R gene allows the in-vitro selection of the marked population so that 100% of the infused cells can be marked; it also allows later in-vitro selection of the marked cells recovered from the patient. This ability to select and expand the marked cell population means that the functional properties of the labeled cells can be assessed after in-vivo selection.

This protocol (Rosenberg et al., 1990b) is open to adult patients with metastatic melanoma in whom all available therapy has failed and who have an expected survival of less than six months. The first 30 to 60 days of the protocol involve the in-vitro culture, transduction, expansion, and safety analysis of TIL that were grown from a resected tumor deposit. Once the patient's TIL cultures are growing well, one-third to one-half of the culture is transduced with the replication-defective neo^R retroviral vector LNL6. Over the following days to weeks, the transduced and nontransduced cultures are grown, expanded, characterized, and subjected to a series of safety assessments. After the cultures are sufficiently expanded and characterized, a mixture of transduced and nontransduced cells is reinfused into the patient. The patients then receive intravenous IL-2 every eight hours for up to five days. Patients are followed by analyzing peripheral blood and tumor biopsies for the presence and persistence of the gene-modified TIL.

The results from the first five patients treated under this protocol have been reported (Rosenberg et al., 1990a). According to all criteria, including the absence of infectious virus in cultured TIL or patients, the procedure was safe. All five patients tolerated the procedure well and no side-effects due to gene transduction were observed. Based on southern blot analysis and enzymatic assays, TIL from all five of the patients contained and expressed the neo^R gene. Cells from four of the patients were successfully grown in high concentrations of G418, a neomycin analog that is toxic to eukaryotic cells unless inactivated by the neo^R gene. PCR analysis consistently demonstrated gene-modified cells in the circulation of all five patients for at least three weeks, and as long as two months in two patients. From the standpoint of TIL trafficking studies, it was of particular interest that gene-modified cells were recovered from tumor deposits of selected patients as many as 64 days after infusion. It has also been possible to select and culture the gene-marked TIL recovered five days after reinfusion from a tumor biopsy (Aebersold, Kasid and Rosenberg, 1990). These studies clearly demonstrated the feasibility of using retroviruses to transfer and express genes in human lymphocytes.

In addition to the ongoing trial at the NCI, two similar trials of neo^R-marked TIL are now under way. In a trial under the direction of M.C. Favrot at the Centre Leon Berard, Lyon, France, TIL cells from metastatic melanoma and renal cell carcinoma are marked with the LNL6 vector (Favrot et al., 1992).

Table 9.3. *Dual marking of TIL and PBL subsets*

Subgroup	Number of patients	Effective cells	Vector	Biological*
A	5	Bulk TIL	LNL6	IL-2
		Bulk PBL	G1Na	
B	5	CD8+ TIL	LNL6	IL-2
		CD8+ PBL	G1Na	
C	5	CD4+ TIL	LNL6	IL-2
		CD4+ PBL	G1Na	
D	5	CD8+ TIL	LNL6	IL-2
		CD4+ PBL	G1Na	

*For renal cell carcinoma interferon-α (IFN-α) also given. Adapted with permission from Economou et al. (1992).

The only differences between this trial and the NCI trial are the inclusion of patients with renal cell carcinoma and the schedule of IL-2 administration. After a five-day IL-2 pretreatment and a six-day rest period, the marked TIL are reinfused, followed by five days of continuous IL-2 infusion, two days of rest, and then six weeks of subcutaneous IL-2 infusion. It is hoped that the predosing and extended dosing with IL-2 may facilitate the intratumoral grafting of the TIL and also improve TIL survival.

More recently, a TIL-marking trial was initiated at the UCLA School of Medicine, Los Angeles, California, under the direction of J. Economou (Economou et al., 1992). This trial was approved for 20 patients with metastatic melanoma and 20 patients with metastatic renal cell carcinoma. Patients will be treated with various combinations of six different cell effector populations: bulk TIL, CD8+ TIL, CD4+ TIL, bulk peripheral blood lymphocyte (PBL), CD8+ PBL, or CD4+ PBL. Subgroups of five patients will receive different combinations of two cellular effectors (Table 9.3). The two cell-effector populations will be marked with different neo[R] vectors, LNL6 or G1Na, that can be distinguished by PCR. After infusion of the two marked cell populations, DNA from peripheral blood, tumor biopsies, and normal tissue will be isolated at various times. PCR using LNL6- or G1Na-specific primers will allow the determination of the relative ratio of each marked cell population in blood, tumor, and normal tissue (Figure 9.1). This marking study will address important questions about TIL, TIL subset, PBL, and PBL subset trafficking, tumor localization, and in-vivo lifespan.

The above-mentioned trials are all gene marker trials. The *neo*[R] gene serves no therapeutic purpose but only serves to aid in-vivo cell trafficking and survival studies. The success of the first TIL gene-marking trial and the

(a)

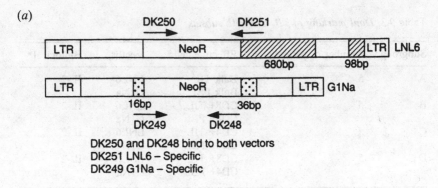

(b)

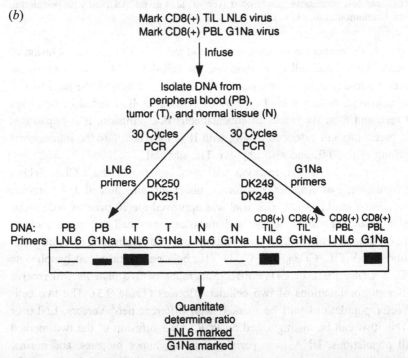

Fig. 9.1. Dual marking with LNL6 and G1Na neo[R] vectors. (a) Diagram of the two neo[R] vectors. Unshaded parts are sequences common to both vectors; right-handed slant sequences are unique to LNL6; dotted pattern sequences are unique to G1Na. Small arrows represent PCR primers. A 790 base pair neo[R]-hybridization probe is made using DK250 and DK248. (b) Diagram of how the ratio of LNL6- to G1Na-marked cells is determined for subgroup B in UCLA TIL trial. Sensitivity and accuracy of method determined by Miller et al. (1992).

finding of marked TIL in tumor biopsies have been logically extended in an attempt to produce locally high concentrations of therapeutic proteins in the tumor via transduction of TIL with a potentially therapeutic gene. The first such TIL gene therapy trial involves the insertion and expression of the gene for TNF in TIL (Rosenberg et al., 1990c). The objective of the trial is to evaluate the toxicity and possible therapeutic efficacy of administering TIL that have been transduced with the gene coding for TNF. Although the exact mechanisms of TNF antitumor effects are not clear, TNF is believed to affect tumor vasculature, and when bound to membranes it also may be involved in direct tumor lysis. TNF has shown great promise in a variety of established experimental murine cancers. However, extensive tests of systematically delivered TNF in humans with advanced cancer have been disappointing in that no antitumor effects were observed. The lack of antitumor effect is believed to be because the maximum tolerated dose (MTD) of TNF in humans is only 2% of the TNF dose required to mediate an antitumor effect in murine models. When high local concentrations of TNF have been achieved in humans via direct intralesional injection or isolated limb perfusion, tumor regressions have been observed. This has led to the hypothesis that TIL modified to produce large amounts of TNF would produce a high local concentration of TNF at the tumor capable of eliciting an antitumor effect without systemic TNF toxicity. The TNF-modified TIL are expected to have enhanced antitumor activity compared to unmodified TIL.

This is a rather controversial trial because TNF has been very poorly expressed by TIL cells, and TNF-modified TIL (TIL_{TNF}) may have lost their ability to target to tumor deposits (Anderson, 1992). The trial is designed as an escalating-dose study with the objective of finding the maximum dose of TIL_{TNF} that can be tolerated by at least 80% of patients. Since the MTD of TIL_{TNF} may be lower than that of unmodified TIL, the initial number of TIL_{TNF} is a dose 30- to 60-fold lower than the MTD of unmodified TIL. After dose escalation of cell number, there will be another phase of TNF-dose escalation resulting from infusing G418-selected TIL_{TNF}. The G418-selected cultures should be 100% TIL_{TNF} rather then between 1% and 11%, as observed in unselected cultures. Again, there will be a dose-escalation phase, with the first dose of G418-selected TIL_{TNF} being 10% of the TIL_{TNF} MTD. Finally, the dose of IL-2 will be escalated. Detailed studies of toxicity as well as possible therapeutic effects will be made. As the TNF vector also contains the *neo*[R] gene, detailed studies of the survival and distribution of the TIL_{TNF} can also be conducted.

Summary

The early results from the first gene-marking trial were very encouraging. No side-effects due to retroviral-mediated gene marking were noted in the first patients treated with neo^R-marked TIL. Similar safety findings have been reported by all other early reports from trials using retroviral vectors for gene marking or gene therapy. The benefits of retroviral-marking technology to lifespan and trafficking studies were clearly demonstrated. The results from the TIL-marking trials should allow optimization of TIL homing to tumor sites. Enhanced TIL homing via either improved cytokine administration protocols or the infusion of selected TIL subsets may directly improve the efficacy and safety of all TIL immunotherapies. Further, possibly dramatic, improvements in antitumor efficacy may result from the successful expression of therapeutic genes in tumor-homing TIL.

Autologous bone marrow transplantation

There is currently a tremendous effort in oncology to maximize the potential of existing chemotherapeutic agents by dose escalation followed by a bone marrow transplant. A major premise behind the upsurge in bone marrow transplantation is that it allows dose intensification of chemotherapy and radiotherapy beyond their usual hematopoietic dose-limiting toxicity, and that these high-dose regimens will cure a greater number of patients than do conventional therapies. Because many chemotherapy drugs have steep tumoricidal dose—response curves, doubling the drug dose may increase tumor cell kill by as much as ten times. Bone marrow transplants make it possible to increase drug doses as much as four-fold to ten-fold over standard doses; therefore it is apparent that bone marrow transplantation after high-dose therapy holds much promise for improving long-term response and cure rates. This high-dose chemotherapy/ABMT strategy is increasingly used in the treatment of marrow-derived malignancies, such as leukemia, as well as of nonmarrow-derived tumors, such as neuroblastoma and metastatic breast cancer.

ABMT are more commonly performed than human leucocyte antigen (HLA)-matched allogeneic bone marrow transplants (AlloBMT) because HLA-matched donors are not usually available and there is a greater risk of transplant-related morbidity and mortality associated with AlloMBT. Although transplant-related mortality is higher with AlloBMT, the overall survival from the two types of transplant is similar because the relapse rate for ABMT is higher than that of AlloBMT. Two alternative, opposing, explanations have been proposed to explain the higher relapse rate from ABMT over AlloBMT.

One explanation is that alloreactive T lymphocytes present in the allogeneic graft play a major role in recognizing and eliminating residual disease in the host. Since these alloreactive T cells are not present in autologous marrow, higher relapse rates would be expected following ABMT. This reasoning suggests that more effort should be directed at eradicating residual disease in the host before autologous transplant. The alternative explanation for increased relapse rates is that the autologous marrow, even though it is harvested during clinical remission, contains residual malignant cells capable of contributing to relapse. This explanation suggests that more effort should be made to purge the autologous marrow of residual malignant cells. It is likely that both mechanisms occur and contribute to relapse, but the relative contribution of each mechanism in any disease or patient remains a very important issue to resolve. Gene marking can be invaluable in resolving these issues.

Marking of marrow and peripheral blood stem cells (PBSC) can also address many fundamental questions about the biology of autologous marrow reconstitution. For example, do autologous marrow grafts contain viable stem cells that reconstitute the patient, or does the autograft only provide a temporary bridge of committed progenitor cells, allowing surviving host stem cells gradually to repopulate the patient? Successful stem cell marking could answer this and many other questions about normal stem cell biology and the biology of autologous reconstitution. This knowledge could allow significant decreases in the morbidity and mortality associated with ABMT. Such improvements could facilitate even more ABMTs, either to larger patient populations or perhaps as repeated transplants to the same patient, allowing multiple courses of high-dose chemotherapy and a better chance for cure.

There are at least 16 ongoing clinical trials using neo^R-marked bone marrow cells. Their purpose is to study the origin of tumor relapse, to study basic issues in ABMT, and to help assess the safety of retroviral-mediated gene transfer. The patients enrolled in these trials have been treated with various chemotherapies and radiotherapies to induce clinical remission, at which time their bone marrow has been harvested and frozen. There are strict eligibility requirements for the minimum marrow harvest, and only a portion of the marrow may be transduced with the neo^R marker. These standards allow sufficient untransduced marrow to be available in case there is any problem in the transduction, and also allows the patient to withdraw from the study at any time before reinfusion.

The first of these bone marrow-marking trials was started at St Jude Children's Research Hospital, Memphis, Tennessee, under the direction of Malcolm Brenner in September of 1991. This trial was a gene-marking trial of ABMT in children in first remission from acute myeloblastic leukemia

(AML) (Brenner et al., 1991). The trial had four main objectives: to estimate at two years the continuous complete remission rate for children with AML in first complete remission who are treated with autologous bone marrow transplant; to determine whether residual malignant cells in the autologous transplant are a source of relapse after ABMT for AML; to determine if autografting after intensified chemotherapy is likely to increase the cure rate for AML; and to study the mechanisms of autologous graft reconstitution. Owing to the poor prognosis of AML, even after ABMT, it is expected that up to 55% of patients will relapse within two years.

Three informative outcomes with different clinical implications were predicted if the patients relapsed (Brenner et al., 1991). *Outcome 1.* Most of the relapse patients have no marked cells, but occasionally patients relapse with monoclonally marked cells. This implies that patients receiving remission marrow do in fact occasionally receive malignant cells and that relapse is monoclonal. There is a low probability of detection of this outcome. *Outcome 2.* Most relapse patients contain both marked and unmarked tumor cells. The provirus integration site may be polyclonal. This implies the marrow contains a number of cells capable of contributing to relapse. *Outcome 3.* The relapsed cells are either monoclonal or polyclonal, and the marker has the same integration site in apparently normal cells of other lineages. This implies that in many AML patients the malignant 'stem cell' is a true multipotent progenitor cell that is present in remission marrow. The clinical implication for outcomes 1 and 2 is that purging remission marrow would be worthwhile and should be further explored. If outcome 2 is found, marking of purged marrow would provide an essential methodology for assessing the effectiveness of various purging techniques. Outcome 3 would imply that a significant proportion of AMLs are in fact stem-cell disorders, and that in these patients current chemotherapy and autografting strategies are not likely to increase their survival.

An overview of the AML protocol is shown in Figure 9.2. Bone marrow is harvested during a chemotherapy-induced complete remission. If at least 1×10^8 mononuclear marrow cells/kg are obtained, patients may enroll in the study. Seventy percent of the harvested marrow is processed and frozen as per standard techniques. The remaining marrow is transduced by culturing in LNL6 or G1N vector-containing supernatants. After transduction, a small aliquot of cells is removed for bone marrow stem cell and microbiological assays. The remaining transduced cells are frozen. The patient will then undergo a ten-day course of marrow ablative therapy (busulfan/Cytoxan). Forty-eight hours after the marrow ablative therapy, 1×10^8 marrow cells/kg (30% marked + 70% unmarked) are infused through a central venous catheter.

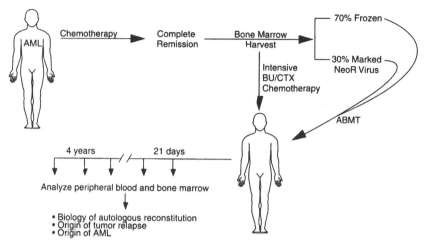

Fig. 9.2. Overview of AML marrow-marking trial. BU/CTX = busulfan/cyclophosphamide; ABMT = autologous bone marrow transplant.

Patient follow-up will include bone marrow aspiration and biopsy on days 21 and 32 post-marrow infusion. Patients will undergo physical examination, complete blood counts, and bone marrow aspiration every six months for the first two years and annually for the next two years. Analysis will include FACS separation and sorting of peripheral blood samples into granulocytes, monocytes, T cells, and B cells. Sorted populations will be analyzed for the neomarker gene insertion to address the mechanisms of autologous reconstitution and the ability to transfect pluripotent stem cells.

A report on the first 20 AML and neuroblastoma patients who have received neo[R]-marked autologous marrow has been published (Brenner et al., 1993a). Two patients died within 21 days of transplantation from disease progression and sepsis, respectively. In the remaining 18 patients, engraftment results were essentially identical to those reported for patients receiving unmodified marrow. These data demonstrate that gene marking does not damage or prevent engraftment by unmodified marrow. The results also suggest that the autologous transplants made substantial contributions to marrow reconstitution. Both patients who have been followed up still had G418-resistant hematopoietic cells at 18 months post-transplant, demonstrating the transduction of an early progenitor cell. The progenitor cells were transduced at a much higher rate than was predicted from animal models. The reason for the higher transduction rate is unknown, but investigators theorize that the extensive chemotherapy these children have undergone may have led to a higher number of cycling progenitor cells that may favor retroviral integration.

Twelve AML patients have been transplanted with neo^R-transduced marrow at St Jude's since September 1991. Two of these 12 patients subsequently relapsed, and in both cases, greater than 2% of the resurgent blast cells contained the neomycin-resistance gene marker (Brenner et al., 1993b). The presence of the neo^R marker was demonstrated by Southern blot analysis of PCR-amplified DNA and by growth of purified blasts in the presence of G418. Patient 1 had two markers uniquely and invariably expressed by the malignant cell population. It was possible to show that this same cell population was present and marked in remission marrow and that progeny of these marked cells formed 2% of the clonogenic cells detected at relapse. These data demonstrate that malignant cells capable of contributing to relapse may be present in autologous marrow harvested from AML patients in apparent complete clinical remission. Although residual disease in the patient may also contribute to disease relapse, these data suggest that effective marrow purging is needed to improve long-term survival after autologous bone marrow transplantation for AML. Similar results have been obtained in the St Jude neuroblastoma trials, where three out of three relapsed patients have neo^R-marked tumors (Rill et al., 1994).

Conventional technologies did not allow the relative efficacy of various purging methods to be ranked since, by definition, even before purging, the marrow had no detectable malignant cells. Before gene marking it was only a matter of belief that the benefits of purging outweigh the damage to normal progenitor cells. Results of the St Jude marrow-marking trials indicate the need for marrow purging in therapies for both AML and neuroblastoma. For AML, a marrow-purging trial comparing the efficacy of 4-hydroxyperoxy-cyclophosphamide (4HC) or IL-2 has opened (Brenner et al., 1994). In a trial of 35 patients, marrow will be harvested, and two different neo^R vectors, LNL6 and G1N, will be used to mark separate one-third aliquots of the collected marrow. The marked marrow will then be randomized and purged with either 4HC or IL-2. After purging, both marrows will be reinfused. If the patient relapses, and the relapse is marked, then the relapse can be associated with a particular purging technique. In this way, relatively small trials can rapidly assess the efficacy of various purging techniques since efficacy would be assessed by absence of a marked relapse rather than an effect on survival or a decrease in relapse rate. A similar dual-vector trial assessing an ex-vivo immunomagnetic purging technique is ongoing for neuroblastoma (Brenner et al., 1993c).

Joyce O'Shaughnessy, Cynthia Dunbar, and their colleagues at the National Institutes of Health (NIH), Bethesda, Maryland, recently initiated trials with multiple myeloma and metastatic breast cancer patients (O'Shaughnessy et al., 1993; Dunbar et al., 1993). A similar trial with chronic myelocytic leukemia (CML) patients will be starting soon. In these trials two different neo^R vectors, LNL6 and GINa, are used to follow separately the fate of marked cells derived from peripheral blood or bone marrow. The breast cancer trial has four main objectives: to study the feasibility of engrafting retrovirally transduced hematopoietic stem cells after high-dose chemotherapy; to study the trafficking and survival times of marked bone marrow and PBSC in both the marrow and peripheral blood during marrow engraftment after high-dose chemotherapy; to study, after bone marrow engraftment, the effects of chemotherapy on the neo^R-marked stem cells and their marked progeny; to study the effects of administered hematopoietic growth factors on the neo^R-marked bone marrow and peripheral blood cells. This series of trials will allow the comparison of the effect of various preparative chemotherapy regimens on engraftment and transduction efficiencies.

Three aspects of the retroviral transduction procedures used in these NIH studies were unique among the human transfer studies conducted to date. These techniques, all designed to increase the efficiency of gene transfer into human stem cells, are the transduction of the CD34+ subpopulation of marrow and peripheral blood cells, the addition of hematopoietic growth factors (IL-3, IL-6, or stem cell factor) to the transduction culture, and a transduction period of two to six days. Since the pluripotent stem cells responsible for short-term and probably long-term marrow reconstitution are believed to express the CD34 antigen, and since most tumor cells do not express CD34, enrichment for CD34+ cells should result in the depletion of any tumor cells contaminating the marrow or peripheral blood, and a reduction in the volume of cells that must be transduced, cryopreserved, and reinfused. The small transduction volume allows a theoretical increase in the multiplicity of infection in the transduction and should reduce complications resulting from the infusion of cellular debris and freezing solutions. As in the St Jude trials, the patients will be extensively pretreated with chemotherapy that may increase the number and cycling of stem cells. These patients will also receive granulocyte macrophage colony stimulating factor (GM-CSF) or granulocyte colony stimulating factor (G-CSF) – treatments that may also serve to increase the number and cycling of stem cells and thus increase the transduction efficiency of pluripotent stem cells.

The breast cancer trial is schematically depicted in Figure 9.3. Patients with metastatic breast cancer will receive four to nine cycles of preinduction chemotherapy to induce at least a partial response (PR). During the preinduction chemotherapy, GM-CSF or G-CSF will be administered to stimulate bone marrow recovery. At least two weeks after the recovery of blood counts following the last cycle of induction chemotherapy, PBSC will be mobilized

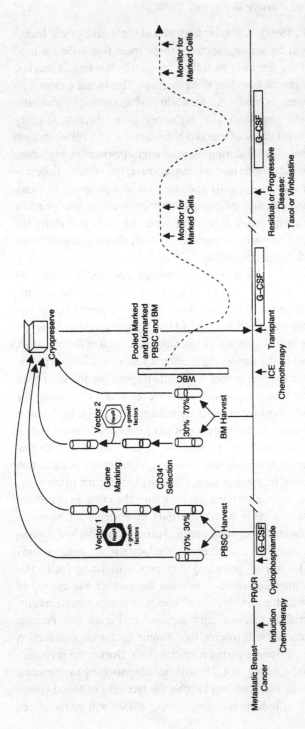

Fig. 9.3. Overview of NIH breast cancer ABMT trial using CD34-selected peripheral blood stem cells (PBSC) and bone marrow (BM). WBC, white blood count; PR/CR, partial response/complete response; G-CSF, granulocyte colony stimulating factor; ICE, ifosfamide, carboplatin, etoposide. (Adapted with permission from Dunbar and Nienhuis, 1993.)

and harvested by apheresis. Two weeks after white blood counts and platelets recover from apheresis, bone marrow will be harvested. Seventy percent of the PBSC and bone marrow will be directly cryopreserved. The remaining 30% of the PBSC and bone marrow will be separately enriched for CD34+ cells using an anti-CD34 antibody and an immunoabsorption column. The PBSC CD34+ cells will be transduced with either the LNL6 or G1N.40 neo^R vector. The bone marrow CD34+ cells will be transduced with the other neo^R vector. Following high-dose ICE chemotherapy (ifosfamide, carboplatin, etoposide), the neo^R-transduced and unmodified PBSC and marrow will be reinfused. Serial peripheral blood and bone marrow samples will be obtained to follow the persistence of neo^R-marked cells and the time course of marrow recovery. Bone marrow and sites of tumor relapse will be biopsied and tested for the presence of the neo^R gene by PCR. Investigators do not expect to find any marked breast cancer cells. The presence of marked breast cancer cells would have serious contraindications for other studies in which chemoprotective genes will be inserted into autologous marrow of breast cancer patients.

After ABMT, patients with residual or progressive disease will be treated with vinblastine or Taxol and with G-CSF. This subset of patients will be studied to determine if a chemotherapy-induced hematopoietic nadir will increase the number of neo^R-marked progenitor and cycling stem cells. In a similar manner, the effect of G-CSF on the number of neo^R-marked bone marrow or circulating cells in the post-nadir recovery period will be examined.

Recently, a trial headed by A. Deisseroth at the M. D. Anderson Cancer Center has begun in which the MDR-1 (multidrug resistance) cDNA is inserted into CD34+ stem cells of ovarian patients undergoing ABMT (Deisseroth, Kavanagh and Champlin, 1994). It is hoped that the MDR-1-modified cells will be resistant to subsequent chemotherapy and therefore be selected for in vivo by cyclical Taxol therapy. The investigators hope that as the MDR-1-transduced hematopoietic cells increase with Taxol selection, the tolerated dose of Taxol will also rise. It is hoped that higher chemotherapy doses can be tolerated after MDR-1 transduction and that the higher doses of chemotherapy will have beneficial effects on patient survival. The same investigators have a similar trial ongoing for breast cancer patients. Several other groups are studying MDR-1 transduction of stem cells.

Summary

Most gene-marker clinical protocols in oncology involve the marking of autologous bone marrow or PBSC by retroviral vectors. The number of protocols reflects both the wide use of ABMT in oncology and the broad range of unanswered fundamental questions about the biology of autologous marrow reconstitution. The early results of these trials validate the theory that the relatively few malignant cells in remission marrow can be marked, and that the large growth amplication of the malignant population that occurs at relapse allows the marking signal to be readily detected if the marked cells do indeed contribute to relapse (Brenner et al., 1993b). Preliminary reports from these marking trials have substantiated the need for marrow purging in therapies for both AML and neuroblastoma. Gene marking will be able rapidly to assess in relatively small trials the efficacy of various purging techniques. Also ongoing are gene therapy trials in which CD34+ cells will be transduced with the *MDR-1* gene, in the hope of protecting the patient from chemotherapy-induced cytopenia, and using subsequent chemotherapy to select in vivo for transduced cells. The ABMT trials are likely to reveal much about the biology of marrow reconstitution. It is likely that these studies will further optimize ABMT procedures, possibly resulting in dramatic reductions in morbidity and mortality. These optimizations have significant implications for both oncology patients and patients with marrow-associated genetic deficiencies such as adenosine deaminase deficiency.

Allogeneic and autologous tumor cell vaccines

In addition to the TIL trials already discussed, many other trials are directed towards use of patients' immune systems to attack their cancer. In these trials, tumor cells are modified to express a variety of genes to enhance the immune response to established tumors (Table 9.4). In preclinical studies it was found that mice, immunized with nonimmunogenic tumor cells transfected with cytokine or major histocompatibility (MHC) genes, are able to reject the gene-modified tumors. Significantly, after the gene-modified tumor vaccinations, the immune system can subsequently also reject unmodified tumor cells. Furthermore, the direct production of cytokines by tumor cells was found to be safer and more efficacious than intralesional cytokine injection.

In numerous trials, the effect of allogeneic and autologous tumor cell vaccines is being studied. A comparison of three different gene therapy approaches to melanoma vaccine development is shown in Figure 9.4. Both the use of allogeneic tumor cell lines and in-vivo gene transfer have the important advantage that they obviate the need to generate an autologous tumor cell line from every patient.

Table 9.4. *Allogeneic and autologous tumor vaccines*

Target cell	Delivery	Cancer	Gene	Retrovirus	Liposome	Adenovirus	Other
Allogeneic tumor cells	Ex vivo	Melanoma	IL-2	2	1		
		Melanoma	IL-4	1			
		Melanoma	IL-2 + IFN	1			
		Melanoma	HLA-B7		1		
		RCC	IL-2	1			
Autologous fibroblasts	Ex vivo	Various	IL-2, IL-4, IL-12	4			
Autologous tumor	Ex vivo	Various	GM-CSF	5			
		Various	HLA-B7		1		
		Ovarian	HSV TK	1			
		Various	Cytokine	10	5		3
Autologous tumor	In vivo	Colorectal	CEA				1
		Various	HLA-B7		8		
		Various	IL-2	1		2	

IL, interleukin; IFN, interferon; HLA-B7, human leucocyte antigen-B7; GM-CSF, granulocyte macrophage colony stimulating factor; HSV TK, herpes simplex virus thymidine kinase; CEA, carcinoembryonic antigen; RCC, renal cell carcinoma.

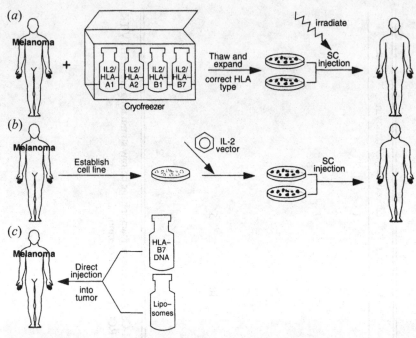

Fig. 9.4. Three gene therapy approaches to melanoma vaccine development. (*a*) Allogeneic vaccines. A bank of well-characterized melanoma cell lines representing various HLA types is created, transduced with IL-2, and frozen. As needed, cells of appropriate HLA type are thawed and expanded. After lethal irradiation, the IL-2-secreting allogeneic cells are injected into the patient to elicit a strong immune response to melanoma-associated antigens. The immune response is to the injected allogeneic cells and to the patient's own unmodified melanoma cells. (b) and (c) Autologous vaccines. (*b*) An autologous cell line is established and transduced for every patient. Transduced cells are injected back into the patient to elicit a strong immune response to both modified and unmodified melanoma cells. (*c*) DNA from a major histocompatibility antigen that is different from that of the patient is mixed with liposomes and injected directly into the tumor. The liposome delivers the *MHC* gene to the tumor cells, making them highly immunogenic. The immune response to the modified cells also recognizes unmodified tumor cells.

Allogeneic irradiated cancer vaccines

There are several ongoing trials using HLA-A2-matched allogeneic tumor cells that have been genetically modified to secrete IL-2. These trials involve metastatic melanoma and metastatic renal cell carcinoma patients. Both cancers are considered good targets for immunotherapy because rare, spontaneous regressions have been observed. These well-documented, spontaneous regressions are believed to result from a strong immune response to the tumor. Furthermore, infusion of IL-2 has been somewhat effective in both cancers, although the effectiveness of direct IL-2 therapy is limited by high systemic toxicity. Theoretically, transduction of tumor cells with IL-2 will achieve the same or better immune stimulation without any systemic toxicity. HLA-matched allogeneic cells were chosen over autologous tumor cells because of the extended time, high cost, and high failure rate in establishing autologous cell lines from every patient. If allogeneic cell lines are effective, then a small series of cell lines representing the various HLA types could be made to treat every patient with a particular cancer.

One such trial is being conducted at University Hospital, Leiden, Netherlands, by S. Osanto and colleagues (Osanto et al., 1993). The objective is to immunize HLA-A1-positive or HLA-A2-positive patients with HLA-A1, A2, B8 allogeneic melanoma cells that have been transfected with a plasmid containing a constitutively expressed IL-2 gene. It is hoped that the immunizations will induce or augment a specific antitumor cytotoxic T lymphocyte response to autologous tumor cells. The investigators will evaluate the toxicity and antitumor efficacy of weekly subcutaneous injections of irradiated allogeneic melanoma cells; investigate any correlation of toxicity or antitumor effects with HLA Class I expression of the patients' metastatic tumor cells and with the cellular infiltrate; and assess induction or strengthening of cellular immunity in responding patients. Immunization will be done weekly for three consecutive weeks. Dosages of irradiated IL-2-producing allogeneic cells will be escalated in consecutive groups of five to ten patients from 6×10^7 cells/week to 1.8×10^8 cells/week. Various immunological tests will be performed on blood, accessible tumors, vaccination site biopsies, and any TIL cells present in tumor biopsies. It is interesting to note that in this early trial the patients are to be hospitalized during the three-week treatment owing to specific concerns the Governmental Recombinant DNA Committee had about the possibility of environmental contamination with engineered DNA!

If no regressions are seen during the first three weeks of immunization in the first group of patients, then these patients will receive low-dose IL-2 on an outpatient basis during the next three weeks. If after six weeks (three weeks with allogeneic cell injections plus three weeks of low-dose IL-2) there are still no regressions, then the low-dose IL-2 pilot will be discontinued. If a patient has a complete or partial remission during the three-week treatment, booster injections of the allogeneic cells will be given every two weeks for up to three consecutive months or until progression of the disease.

B. Gansbacher is directing two pilot studies of allogeneic cancer vaccines at Memorial Sloane-Kettering Cancer Center, New York City, New York (Gansbacher et al., 1992a, 1992b). One trial is for metastatic melanoma and the other is for renal cell carcinoma. Both of these trials involve the use of cell lines that were transduced with IL-2 retroviral vectors. They are dose-escalation trials involving two possible doses. Ten million irradiated, allogeneic tumor cells will be injected in the low-dose group; 50 million irradiated cells will be injected in the high-dose group. Each patient should receive a vaccination on days 1, 15, 29, and 85. If the patient has a complete or partial response, additional booster injections will be given every three months for one year or until disease progression. Like the Osanto trial, these two trials are testing irradiated allogeneic tumor cells that express IL-2. The major differences are that a much lower total number of cells will be injected, and no supplemental doses of IL-2 will be provided. Patients will be followed for antitumor response, immunological response to the treatment, and any evidence of exposure to replication-competent virus.

Autologous cancer vaccines

Other trials are studying the potential antitumor activity of vaccines derived from the patients' own tumor cells. Some trials require the establishment of a tumor cell line from each patient with subsequent in-vitro gene transduction. After gene modification, the cells are returned to the patient via a subcutaneous or intradermal injection. The modified tumor cells are not irradiated before injection but are not expected to grow, since the transduced gene should make them highly immunogenic. As an additional safety measure, if the injected cells do grow, they will be surgically removed and the site of injection treated by local irradiation. Also, patient eligibility requires that the patient already has a large tumor burden compared to the number of injected cells. Other autologous cancer vaccine trials are using in-vivo gene delivery, so no cell lines are required.

A straightforward Phase I study of the ability of a vaccination with IL-2-transduced neuroblastoma cells to alter disease progression of relapsed neuro-blastoma has been initiated at St Jude Children's Research Hospital (Brenner et al., 1992). Children eligible for this trial must have already failed autologous bone marrow transplantation, have measurable disease, and have a transduced cell line available that produces $\geq$150 pg IL-2/10^6 cells per 24 hours. It is expected that after the completion of this immunotherapy, the patients will be entered into other ongoing Phase I or II studies of conventional agents. The trial has three objectives: to determine the safety of two weekly subcutaneous injections of IL-2-transduced autologous neuroblastoma cells; to determine whether major histocompatibility antigen (MHC)-restricted or unrestricted antitumor immune responses are induced by the subcutaneous injections and the cell dose needed to produce these effects; and to obtain preliminary data

Table 9.5. *Dose escalation of IL-2/neuroblastoma cells*

Level	Dose day 1 (tumor cells/kg)	Dose day 8 (tumor cells/kg)
1	10^5	10^6
2	10^6	10^7
3	10^7	10^8
4	10^8	10^8

Printed with permission from Brenner et al. (1992).

on the antitumor effects of this approach. The cytokine IL-2 was chosen because there is in-vitro and in-vivo evidence that IL-2 has immunomodulatory effects that would help neuroblastoma patients, and animal models have shown that IL-2 augments tumor immunogenicity across a broad range of tumor types, including the murine neuroblastoma cell line C1300.

This is a dose-escalation Phase I study. Viable cells are used because experiments have shown that neuroblastoma cells die rapidly after irradiation before they can secrete enough IL-2 to generate an in-vivo immune response. Furthermore, a number of investigators dispute the notion that irradiated cells are immunogenic. At least three patients will be admitted at each dosage level until the maximum tolerated dose (MTD) is found (Table 9.5). Patients will be treated with two subcutaneous injections of IL-2-modified tumor cells. The second injection is given one week after the first and will contain ten times more cells than the first injection, up to a maximum of 10^8 tumor cells/kg. After a three-week to four-week rest, the patients will be re-evaluated for evidence of toxicity and response. Responding patients who do not have excessive toxicity can receive up to two additional injections at one-week intervals. The study will end when the MTD has been reached. In addition to the normal toxicity criteria, another toxicity criterion is any evidence of the growth of injected tumor cells confirmed by biopsy. Although the injected cells are viable, they are not expected to grow since the IL-2 modification should make them highly immunogenic.

Follow-up includes punch biopsies of the injection site before the second injection, and another 10−14 days later. Further analysis will be done of blood samples obtained at weekly intervals for six weeks, biweekly intervals for another six weeks, and the monthly for a year. Immunologic changes will be assessed for a year. Long-term analysis of retrovirus or vector content by PCR and reverse transcriptase assays will be done for ten years.

Two trials involving attempts both to immunize the patients to their own tumor as well as to provide a local immunization that can be used to grow lymphocytes for adoptive immunotherapy have been initiated at the Surgery Branch, NCI (Rosenberg et al., 1992a, 1992b). The investigators supervising these two trials are studying the modification of autologous cancer cells with either TNF or IL-2. Three weeks after vaccination, TIL for adoptive immunotherapy will be grown from either the lymph nodes draining the injection site or directly from the modified tumor cells growing in vivo. Both of these trials are open to patients with melanoma, renal cell carcinoma, or colon carcinoma that has metastasized, and who have an expected survival of six months or less, and for whom standard curative and palliative measures have been exhausted. The gene-modified cells should be more immunogenic than the unmodified tumor and should, therefore, improve the efficacy of both the autologous tumor vaccines and subsequent adoptive immunotherapy.

As in the St Jude neuroblastoma protocol, it is necessary to be able to establish and transduce a cell line from each patient. Modified autologous tumor cells, 2×10^8 viable cells, will be injected subcutaneously into the patient's thigh. At the same time, the patient will also receive two intradermal injections of 2×10^7 modified, viable tumor cells about 3 cm from the site of subcutaneous injection. All three sites will be marked with tattoo ink so they can be monitored and subsequently removed. The intradermal injection should result in rapid draining to the lymph nodes. The subcutaneous injections are also done because there is some evidence that better TIL are raised from visceral tumors. After three weeks, the superficial inguinal lymph nodes draining the inoculation site will be removed and TIL grown. Growth of the injected, modified tumor cells is not expected, but if it does occur, when the modified tumor cells reach 1 cm they will be excised and used as a source of TIL cells. If no tumor cell growth is observed eight weeks after injection, then the injection sites will be excised and biopsied for pathologic examination. Cultured lymphocytes will be expanded and used for adoptive immunotherapy, as detailed in previous protocols.

A much easier autologous tumor technology is being pursued by several investigators. A specific example of this type of study is that of Nabel et al. (1992). This trial is quite different from the previously discussed trials because it is using nonviral DNA/liposome complexes instead of retroviral vectors. Another major difference is that the gene transfer is done in vivo. This trial is introducing the highly immunogenic major histocompatibility complex antigen HLA-B7 directly into cutaneous melanoma tumors of non-HLA-B7 patients using DNA/liposome complexes injected directly into tumor nodules. The use of DNA/liposome complexes allows great flexibility in the delivered DNA, there are no constraints on DNA size, and no requirements for viral regulatory elements, which can interfere with the expression of the target

Table 9.6. *Dose escalation of HLA-B7/DC-Chol*

Group	Number of injections per treatment	Volume of injection (ml)	Times of repeated treatment	Total number of treatments
I	1	≤0.2	2 weeks	3
II	3	≤0.2	2 weeks	3
III	5	≤0.2	2 weeks	3
IV	5	≤0.4	2 weeks	4

Printed with permission from Nabel et al. (1992).

gene. Direct in-vivo transduction of tumor cells has several strong benefits over in-vitro methods of cell transduction because there is no need to establish a cell line from each patient. This reduces concerns about the alteration of a tumor's phenotype by growth in vitro, the outgrowth of aberrant transformed cells in culture, and the future cost and general utility of this gene therapy technology. Potential problems include inefficient gene integration and possibly low efficiency of gene transfer.

Preclinical animal studies have demonstrated immune recognition of and protection against established tumors following in-vivo treatment of non-immunogenic tumors. One concern arises from the detection of plasmid DNA in the heart, lung, or kidney of some animals whose tumors were injected with the DNA/liposome complexes (Plautz et al., 1993). However, no evidence of vector DNA has ever been found in the testes or ovaries of any animal, even after intravenous injection of the DNA/liposome complexes. Until the issue of the presence of DNA in nontumor tissue is resolved, the clinical protocol excludes any patient capable of having children (Nable, 1992).

A Phase I dose-escalation trial intended to evaluate the safety and appropriate dosage of DNA/liposome for introducing a recombinant HLA-B7 antigen into human tumors in vivo was started in June 1992. Other objectives included documenting recombinant gene expression in vivo and characterizing the specificity and mechanism of the immune response against the introduced antigen. The study design is as follows. Twelve adult patients with histologically confirmed cutaneous melanoma that is unresponsive to standard treatments, who are negative for HLA-B7, who have an expected survival of one year or less, and who are incapable of having children, are to be studied in a four-group, dose-escalation series (Table 9.6). Each group will be treated sequentially, with at least one month observation prior to dose escalation. Dose escalation will proceed if all three patients show toxicities ≤ grade 3.

Before treatment, serum samples will be drawn from patients. Prior to treatment, the nodule to be injected, as well as some untreated control nodules, will be imaged by computerized tomography (CT) and their sizes determined. Under local anesthetic, a needle biopsy will be performed and then the DNA/liposome will be injected. To assure that the DNA/liposome is not injected intravenously, gentle aspiration will be applied to the syringe prior to injection. Immediately after the injection, a blood sample will be obtained and analyzed by PCR for the presence of plasmid DNA in the peripheral blood. The treatment is repeated three to four times at two-week intervals in patients for whom toxicity is ≤ grade 2. Just before repeat injections, the nodule will be needle biopsied for later analysis. The biopsies will be analyzed for confirmation of gene transfer and expression by PCR and immunohistochemical and/or immunofluorescent staining. Pathologic analysis of the biopsies will also be done. The specific immune response to HLA-B7 will be analyzed using cytolytic T cell assays.

Gary Nabel has reported encouraging preliminary data from the first five patients treated under this protocol. No toxicity has been observed in any of the patients, and expression of the introduced HLA-B7 gene has been observed in post-treatment biopsies from all five patients (personal communication; Nabel et al., 1993).

Nabel's group has closed this initial protocol and replaced it with a protocol containing four technological improvements (Nabel et al., 1994): more efficacious liposomes; an optimized vector that expresses both HLA-B7 and β-2 microglobulin; catheter delivery of the DNA/liposome to the tumor; and application to several types of cancer. The new protocol is also designed to examine the therapeutic effect of adding IL-2 into some treatment regimens. Similar protocols using the same cationic liposome and DNA are under way at several sites for several different cancers.

Summary

There are currently three different gene-therapy approaches to the development of cancer vaccines (see Figure 9.4). All three approaches have demonstrated promising results in animal models. Currently it is unclear which are the best genes for augmenting tumor immunogenicity due to conflicting animal data and because the action of cytokines is often species specific. It is also unclear whether irradiated or nonirradiated cells are better for stimulating tumor rejection. Several small human trials that assess specific immunological parameters may provide some much-needed answers to these and other questions.

It is likely that these vaccines will initially find their greatest utility in helping to eliminate minimal residual disease following surgery, radiation therapy, or chemotherapy. Success with either allogeneic tumor vaccines or the direct in-vivo generation of autologous vaccines would make it easy to develop 'off the shelf reagents' that could be quickly and cost-efficiently provided to large patient populations. Such easy and inexpensive technology would also enable the trial of similar vaccines for cancer prevention.

Suicide, antisense, or tumor suppressor gene delivery to autologous tumors in situ

The previously discussed autologous tumor trials are predicated on the basis of using the immune system to start, maintain, and finish the entire cascade of events needed to cure a patient of his or her cancer. Several, more direct, approaches to cancer therapy are also under very active investigation. These approaches do not disregard the role the immune system can play in destroying tumor cells, but are not focused on using the immune system to start the therapy. They focus on delivery of a gene whose gene product will have an active role in killing the cancer cell by either a chemotherapy-type approach, e.g., a suicide or drug-susceptibility gene, or by inducing apoptosis or differentiation, e.g., via a tumor suppressor gene or an antisense molecule against an oncogene. These methods are targeted to in-situ tumors using in-vivo gene delivery.

One approach is to use retroviral vectors to introduce a drug-sensitivity gene into dividing tumor cells in the in-situ milieu of normal nondividing tissue. This approach exploits a potential drawback of retroviral vectors – their inability to transfer genes into nondividing cells – and turns it into an advantage. Once the dividing tumor cells have been modified, there exists a *qualitative* difference between the tumor and normal cells that can be exploited for selective cancer chemotherapy (Huber, Richards and Austin, 1994). Following gene delivery, systemic administration of a nontoxic prodrug results in drug activation only in the gene-modified cells, i.e., tumor cells. This creates a locally high concentration of an active drug at the tumor site without systemic toxicity.

E. Oldfield is leading a trial at NIH that is implanting herpes simplex virus thymidine kinase (HSV TK) retrovirus vector-producing cells (VPC) directly into brain tumors (Oldfield et al., 1993). The injected cells have been engineered to produce a retroviral vector that carries the HSV TK gene, a drug-susceptibility gene that makes transfected cells sensitive to gancyclovir (GCV). The VPC are delivered by stereotactic injection into the tumor mass where they produce HSV TK retrovirus. The retroviruses are thereby continuously available to infect neighboring proliferating cells until the VPC are rejected by the immune system or are killed by GCV therapy. Since essentially the only proliferating cells in the brain are tumor cells, and to a lesser degree cells establishing tumor vasculature, the tumor and perhaps the tumor vasculature will be selectively made HSV TK positive. Subsequent GCV treatment will kill the cells expressing HSV TK, i.e., the tumor cells and the murine vector-producing cells, but is generally nontoxic to normal, untransduced cells.

Preclinical animal studies suggested that this approach can mediate complete tumor regression without the need for surgical excision, irradiation, or traditional nonspecific chemotherapy. Furthermore, animal studies have demonstrated a neighboring or bystander killing effect wherein complete regression of tumors was observed following GCV treatment of tumors that consisted of 10% HSV TK-modified tumor cells and 90% unmodified, wild-type tumor cells (Culver et al., 1992; Oldfield et al., 1993). The mechanism of this 'bystander tumor kill' is not understood, since it is believed that phosphorylated GCV derivatives are the agents responsible for cell killing and that they should not be diffusible from the tumor cell.

The clinical study has three main objectives: to determine if intratumoral delivery of xenogenic VPC into human brain tumors will result in in-vivo transduction of the tumor; to determine if GCV treatment of the HSV TK-transduced tumor will result in tumor eradication; and to evaluate the short- and long-term consequences of the implantation of xenogenic VPC. Twenty adult patients with malignant brain tumors that have failed all standard therapy will be enrolled. Ten of these patients are expected to have primary brain tumors. The other ten patients will have brain metastases from primary lung cancer, breast cancer, malignant melanoma, or renal cell carcinoma.

Patients will be divided into two groups based on the surgical accessibility of their tumors. Group 1 patients will have lesion(s) in areas that are surgically accessible with acceptable operative risk. These patients will have HSV TK VPC injected into their brain tumor by magnetic resonance imaging (MRI)-guided stereotactic injection. Multiple injections will be done into large tumors. Seven days after VPC injection, a craniotomy will be performed and complete tumor removal attempted. During surgery, the lining of the surgical cavity will be infiltrated at multiple sites with VPC. GCV will be administered for 14 days, starting five days after craniotomy. The surgically removed tumor will be analyzed for murine cells and virus transduction. This group of patients will provide information regarding the efficacy of in-vivo tumor transduction. However, in this group of patients the evaluation of the therapy's biological effect will be limited and delayed by the operative attempt at tumor resection.

Group 2 patients will have surgically inaccessible tumors or an unaccept-

Table 9.7. *In-vivo delivery of suicide, antisense, and tumor suppressor genes*

Gene	Cancer	Retrovirus	Liposome	Adenovirus	Other
HSV TK	Brain	10		2	
	Melanoma	2			
	Mesothelioma			1	
CD	Colorectal			1	
	Breast				1
Antisense	Breast	1			
	Prostate	1			
	Lung	1			
p53	Lung			1	
	Colorectal			1	
	Head and neck			1	
scAb	Ovarian			1	

ably high operative risk. They will have HSV TK VPC injected into their brain tumor by MRI-guided stereotactic injection. Seven days after the stereotactic injection, GCV will be administered for 14 days. This group of patients will provide a direct evaluation of this approach on the tumor size: any change in size should be completely dependent on the efficacy of tumor transduction and GCV treatment.

Since December 1992, eight patients with brain tumors have received intra-tumoral injection, of murine packaging cells and subsequent GCV treatment. Six patients had primary brain tumors and two had metastatic tumors. All eight patients have tolerated the procedure very well. Five of the patients demonstrated antitumor responses. So far there has been a correlation between the dose of injected producer cells and the degree of antitumor response. The investigators are encouraged by their results, but it is too soon to reach any conclusions about efficacy after such a short follow-up and limited number of patients (Randall, 1993; *Businesswire*, 1993). Fourteen similar trials using HSV TK vectors have been initiated or are scheduled to start soon. These trials will add additional elements: repeat administration, pediatric patients, a broader range of tumor types, and other delivery vectors to the earlier studies (Table 9.7).

A trial using the *E. coli* cytosine deaminase gene (*CD*) was approved at the September 1995 Recombinant DNA Advisory Committee (RAC) meeting. In this protocol, R. Crystal of The Rockefeller University Hospital, New

York, plans to use adenoviruses to deliver the *CD* suicide gene to liver metastases of colon cancer. The adenoviruses will be directly injected into a measured tumor nodule on days one and seven. A second uninjected nodule will serve as a control. On days 2–15 the patient will receive the CD prodrug 5-fluorocytosine (5-FC). The 5-FC is converted by CD into 5-fluorouracil (5-FU), the drug of choice for colorectal cancer. Patients undergoing surgery independent of this study will have both the treated and control nodules removed by laparotomy. The removed nodules will be analyzed to assess gene delivery and expression. Patients not undergoing surgery will be studied based on clinical efficacy parameters. The goals of this trial are: to determine the toxicity of direct administration of the $AD_{CV}CD.10$ vector to hepatic metastases in combination with oral 5-FC; to demonstrate in-vivo gene transfer of a therapeutic gene to a human solid tumor using a replication-deficient adenovirus vector; and to determine if CD adenovirus/5-FC therapy results in tumor changes that support further clinical study. Preclinical data supporting this protocol have been published (Hirschowitz et al., 1995). The clinical protocol has been published in *Human Gene Therapy* (Crystal et al., 1997).

Another method of treating primary and metastatic liver tumors is under investigation by A. Venook and R. Warren at the University of California, San Francisco. They are planning to directly infuse adenoviruses expressing the wild-type *p53* tumor suppressor gene into the hepatic artery. The selectivity and safety of this approach result from the regional delivery to the tumor – liver tumors obtain 80% of their blood supply from the hepatic artery, while normal hepatocytes receive most of their blood from the portal vein – and the benign effect wild-type *p53* is expected to have on normal cells. It is hoped that the expression of wild-type *p53* in the tumor will suppress tumor growth or induce apoptosis. Protocols from the M. D. Anderson Cancer Center involving adenoviral delivery of wild-type *p53* to non-small cell lung cancer and head and neck squamous cell carcinoma have also been approved by RAC. One pervading issue during RAC review of these protocols is concern that the adenoviral stocks used in these trials may contain some low, but clinically significant, level of mutated *p53* genes that will be harmful to the patient.

Antisense *c-fos*, and antisense *c-myc* are being delivered to breast and prostate tumors, respectively, using retroviruses that are delivered either directly into the tumor or regionally. The antisense gene is transcribed from the retroviral mouse mammary tumor virus long terminal repeat (MMTV LTR), resulting in selective expression in breast and prostate cells. J. Holt at Vanderbilt University Medical Center, Nashville, Tennessee, has initiated a trial for breast cancer metastatic to the pleural or peritoneal space (Holt et al., 1996). The pleural or peritoneal effusions will be drained and the fluid replaced by retroviral supernatants. Because retroviruses can only infect dividing cells and the majority of the dividing cells in these fluids will be metastatic breast cancer cells, the treatment should preferentially infect the tumor cells. As a further level of safety, the antisense *c-fos* is transcribed from the breast-specific MMTV LTR. The goals of the trial are: to determine if there is effective transfer and expression of the retroviral vector into malignant breast cells; to determine if the MMTV LTR is specifically expressed in breast cells; to determine toxicity associated with retroviral infusions; and to determine if there is an effective reduction in the number of malignant cells in the effusions following retroviral vector therapy. A similar trial by M. Steiner and J. Holt is planned for prostate cancer. This trial will inject MMTV LTR antisense *c-myc* retroviruses directly into prostate tumors.

Summary

The delivery of genes to tumors in situ is an area of increasing study. With the positive reassurance, in regard to safety, gained from the first human gene-transfer studies, the field of human gene therapy is increasingly moving toward in-vivo gene delivery. The scope of effort is also being broadened with regard to the genes being delivered and to the vectors being used. Preclinical studies suggest that suicide gene delivery can effectively treat a large tumor mass and also prime the immune system to recognize unmodified tumor (Mullen et al., 1994). Therefore regional treatments of bulky disease may also lead to control of distant metastases.

Conclusion

So far, all gene marker/therapy trials in oncology have run smoothly, with no untoward or unexpected toxicities or problems. At this time, no side-effects attributable to retroviral vectors or cationic liposomes have been observed. The number of patients who have been treated is growing quickly, but is still too small to determine the absolute safety of gene marking/gene therapy with regard to insertional mutagenesis, improper regulation of inserted genes, etc. However, the relative safety of these methods is being established daily as increasing numbers of patients are treated without any acute toxicity. Exciting insights into bone marrow reconstitution following ABMT and the efficacy of marrow-purging techniques are virtually guaranteed from gene-marking trials. Preliminary results from trials designed to examine in-vivo delivery and expression in tumors that are resected a short time after therapy should be available relatively quickly. Major breakthroughs in cancer therapy will occur if even half of the promising results of preclinical animal models are found in human trials.

References

Aebersold, P., Kasid, A. and Rosenberg, S. A. (1990). Selection of gene-marked tumor infiltrating lymphocytes from post-treatment biopsies: a case study. *Human Gene Therapy*, **1**: 373–84.

Anderson, C. (1992). Gene therapy researcher under fire over controversial cancer trials. *Nature*, **360**: 399–400.

Brenner, M., Mirro, Jr, J., Hurwitz, C., Santana, V., Ihle, J., Krance, R., Ribeiro, R., Roberts, W. M., Mahmoud, H., Schell, M., Garth, K., Moen, R. C. and French-Anderson, W. (1991). Autologous bone marrow transplant for children with AML in first complete remission: use of marker genes to investigate the biology of marrow reconstitution and the mechanism of relapse. *Human Gene Therapy*, **2**: 137–59.

Brenner, M. K., Furman, W. L., Santana, V. M., Bowman, L., Meyer, W., Crist, W. M., Campana, D., Douglass, E. C., Ihle, J., Boyett, J., Hurwitz, J., Rao, B. N., Jenkins, J. J., Fletcher, B., Kaufman, W., Moen, R. and Kuebing, D. (1992). Phase I study of cytokine-modified autologous neuroblastoma cells for the treatment of relapsed/refractory neuroblastoma. *Human Gene Therapy*, **3**: 665–76.

Brenner, M. K., Rill, D. R., Holladay, M. S., Heslop, H. E., Moen, R. C., Buschle, M., Krance, R. A., Santana, V. M., Anderson, W. F. and Ihle, J. N. (1993a). Gene marking to determine whether autologous marrow infusion restores longterm haemopoiesis in cancer patients. *Lancet*, **342**: 1134–7.

Brenner, M. K., Rill, D. R., Moen, R. C., Krance, R. A., Mirro, J., Jr, Anderson, W. F. and Ihle, J. N. (1993b). Gene-marking to trace origin of relapse after autologous bone-marrow transplantation. *Lancet*, **341**: 85–6.

Brenner, M., Santana, V., Bowman, L., Furman, W., Heslop, H., Krance, R., Mahmoud, H., Boyett, J., Moss, T., Moen, R. C. and Mills, B. (1993c). Use of marker genes to investigate the mechanism of relapse and the effect of bone marrow purging in autologous transplantation for stage D neuroblastoma. *Human Gene Therapy*, **4**: 809–20.

Brenner, M., Krance, R., Heslop, H. E., Santana, V., Ihle, J., Ribeiro, R., Roberts, W. M., Mahmoud, H., Boyett, J., Moen, R. C. and Klingemann, H. G. (1994). Assessment of the efficacy of purging by using gene marked autologous marrow transplantation for children with AML in first complete remission. *Human Gene Therapy*, **5**: 481–99.

Businesswire (1993). Genetic therapy reports interim results of brain cancer trial. September 8.

Crystal, R. G. (1995). Transfer of genes to humans: early lessons and obstacles to success. *Science*, **270**: 404–10.

Crystal, R. G., Hershowitz, E. and Lieberman, M. (1997). A phase I study of direct administration of a replication-deficient adenovirus vector containing the *E. coli* cytosine deaminase gene to metastatic colon carcinoma of the liver in association with the oral administration of the pro-drug 5-fluorocytosine. *Human Gene Therapy*, **8**: 985–1001.

Culver, K. W., Ram, Z., Wallbridge, S., Ishii, H., Oldfield, E. H. and Blaese, R. M. (1992). In vivo gene transfer with retroviral vector-producer cells for treatment of experimental brain tumors. *Science*, **256**: 1550–2.

Deisseroth, A. B., Kavanagh, J. and Champlin, R. (1994). Use of safety-modified retroviruses to introduce chemotherapy resistance sequences into normal hemato-poietic cells for chemoprotection during the therapy of ovarian cancer: a pilot study. *Human Gene Therapy*, **5**: 1507–22.

Dunbar, C. E. and Nienhuis, A. W. (1993). Multiple myeloma: new approaches to therapy. *Journal of the American Medical Association*, **269**: 2412–16.

Dunbar, C. E., Nienhuis, A. W., Stewart, F. M., Quesenberry, P., O'Shaughnessy, J., Cowan, K., Cottler-Fox, M., Leitman, S., Goodman, S., Sorrentino, B. P., McDonagh, K. and Young, N. S. (1993). Amendment to clinical research projects. Genetic marking with retroviral vectors to study the feasibility of stem cell gene transfer and the biology of hematopoietic reconstitution after autologous transplantation in multiple myeloma, chronic myelogenous leukemia, or metastatic breast cancer. *Human Gene Therapy*, **4**: 205–22.

Economou, J. S., Figlin, R. A., Jacobs, E., Golub, S., DeKernion, J., Moen, R. C., Belldegrun, A., Holmes, E. C., Kohn, D., Shau, H. and McBridge, W. H. (1992). The treatment of patients with metastatic melanoma and renal cell cancer using in vitro expanded and genetically-engineered (neomycin phosphotransferase) bulk, CD8(+) and/or CD4(+) tumor infiltrating lymphocytes and bulk, CD8(+) and/or CD4(+) peripheral blood leukocytes in combination with recombinant inter-leukin-2 alone, or with recombinant interleukin-2 and recombinant alpha inter-feron. *Human Gene Therapy*, **3**: 411–30.

Favrot, M. C., Philip, T., Merrouche, Y., Negrier, S., Mercatello, A., Coronel, B., Clapisson, G., Lanier, F., Heilman, M. O., Ranchere, J. Y., Philip, I., Moskov-tchenko, J. F., Tolstoshev, P., Moen, R. and Franks, C. R. (1992). Treat-ment of patients with advanced cancer using tumor infiltrating lymphocytes transduced with the gene of resistance to neomycin. *Human Gene Therapy*, **3**: 533–42.

Fisher, B., Packard, B. S., Read, E. J., Carrasquillo, J. A., Carter, C. S., Topalian, S. L., Yang, J. C., Yolles, P., Larson, S. M. and Rosenberg, S. A. (1989). Tumor localization of adoptively transferred indium-111 labeled tumor infiltrating lymphocytes in patients with metastatic melanoma. *Journal of Clinical Oncology*, **7**: 250–61.

Gansbacher, B., Houghton, A., Livingston, P., Minasian, L., Rosenthal, F., Gilboa, E., Golde, D., Oettigen, H., Steffens, T., Yang, S. Y. and Wong, G. (1992a). A pilot study of immunization with HLA-A2 matched allogeneic melanoma cells that secrete interleukin-2 in patients with metastatic melanoma. *Human Gene Therapy*, **3**: 677–90.

Gansbacher, B., Motzer, R., Houghton, A., Bander, N., Minasian, L., Gastl. G., Rosen-thal, F., Gilboa, E. Scheinfeld, J., Yang, S. Y., Wong, G. J., Golde, D., Reuter, V., Livingston, P., Bosel, G., Nanus, D. and Fair, W. R. (1992b). A pilot study of immunization with interleukin-2 secreting allogeneic HLA-A2 matched renal call carcinoma cells in patients with advanced renal cell carcinoma. *Human Gene Therapy*, **3**: 691–703.

Hirschowitz, E. A., Ohwada, A., Pascal, W. R., Russi, T. J. and Crystal, R. G. (1995). In vivo adenovirus-mediated gene transfer of the *Escherichia coli* cytosine deaminase gene to human colon carcinoma-derived tumors induces chemosensi-tivity to 5-fluorocytosine. *Human Gene Therapy*, **6**: 1055–63.

Holt, J., Arteaga, C. B., Robertson, D. and Moses, H. L. (1996). Gene therapy for the treatment of metastatic breast cancer by in vivo transduction with breast-targeted retroviral vector expressing antisense c-fos RNA. *Human Gene Therapy*, **7**: 1367–80.

Huber, B. E., Richards, C. A. and Austin, E. A. (1994). Virus-directed enzyme/prodrug therapy (VDEPT) selectively engineering drug sensitivity into tumors. *Annals of the New York Academy of Sciences*, **716**: 104–14.

Marshall, E. (1995). Gene therapy's growing pains. *Science*, **269**: 1050–55.

Miller, A. D. (1992). Human gene therapy comes of age. *Nature*, **357**: 455–60.

Miller, A. R., Skotzko, M. J., Rhoades, K., Belldegrun, A. S., Tso, C-L., Kaboo, R., McBride, W. H., Jacobs, E., Kohn, D. B., Moen, R. and Economou, J. S. (1992). Simultaneous use of two retroviral vectors in human gene therapy marking trials: feasibility and potential applications. *Human Gene Therapy*, **3**: 619–24.

Morgan, R. A. and Anderson, W. F. (1993). Human gene therapy. *Annual Review of Biochemistry*, **62**: 191–217.

Mullen, C. A., Coale, M. M., Lowe, R. and Blaese, R. M. (1994). Tumors expressing the cytosine deaminase suicide gene can be eliminated in vivo with 5-fluorocytosine and induce protective immunity to wild type tumor. *Cancer Research*, **54**: 1503–06.

Nabel, G. J. (1992). Response to the points to consider for immunotherapy of malignancy by in vivo gene transfer into tumors. *Human Gene Therapy*, **3**: 705–11.

Nabel, G. J., Chang, A., Nabel, E. G., Plautz, G., Fox, B. A., Huang, L. and Shu, S. (1992). Immunotherapy of malignancy by in vivo gene transfer into tumors. *Human Gene Therapy*, **3**: 399–410.

Nabel, G. J., Nabel, E. G., Yang, Z., Fox, B. A., Plautz, G. E., Gao, X., Huang, L., Shu, S., Gordon, D. and Chang, A. E. (1993). Direct gene transfer with DNA liposome complexes: expression and lack of toxicity in human melanoma. *Proceedings of the National Academy of Sciences of the United States of America*, **90**: 11307–11.

Nabel, G. J., Nabel, E. G., Yang, Z., Fox, B. A., Plautz, G. E., Gao, X., Huang, L., Shu, S., Gordon, D. and Chang, A. E. (1994). Clinical protocol: Immunotherapy for cancer by direct gene transfer into tumors. *Human Gene Therapy*, **5**: 57–77.

Oldfield, E. H., Ram, Z., Culver, K. W., Blaese, R. M., DeVroom, H. L. and Anderson, W. F. (1993). Gene therapy for the treatment of brain tumors using intra-tumoral transduction with the thymidine kinase gene and intravenous ganciclovir. *Human Gene Therapy*, **4**: 39–69.

Osanto, S., Brouwenstÿn, N., Vaessen, N., Figdor, C. G., Melief, C. J. M. and Schrier, P. I. (1993). Immunization with interleukin-2 transfected melanoma cells. A phase I–II study in patients with metastatic melanoma. *Human Gene Therapy*, **4**: 323–30.

O'Shaughnessy, J. A., Cowan, K. H., Wilson, W., Bryant, G., Goldspiel, B., Gress, R., Nienhuis, A. W., Dunbar, C., Sorrentino, B., Stewart, F. M., Moen, R., Fox, M. and Leitman, S. (1993). Pilot study of high dose ICE (ifosfamide, carboplatin, etoposide) chemotherapy and autologous bone marrow transplant (ABMT) with neoR-transduced bone marrow and peripheral blood stem cells in patients with metastatic breast cancer. *Human Gene Therapy*, **4**: 331–54.

Plautz, G. E., Yang, Z-Y., Wu, B-Y., Gao, X., Huang, L. and Nabel, G. J. (1993). Immunotherapy of malignancy by in vivo gene transfer into tumors. *Proceedings of the National Academy of Sciences of the United States of America*, **90**: 4645–9.

Randall, T. (1993). Gene therapy for brain tumors in trials, correction of inherited disorders a hope. *Journal of the American Medical Association*, **269**: 2181–2.

Rill, D. R., Santana, V. M., Roberts, M., Nilson, T., Bowman, L. C., Krance, R. A., Heslop, H. E., Moen, R. C., Ihle, J. N. and Brenner, M. K. (1994). Direct demonstration that autologous bone marrow transplantation for solid tumors can return a multiplicity of tumorigenic cells. *Blood*, **84**: 380–3.

Rosenberg, S. A., Packard, B. S., Aebersold, P. M., Solomon, D., Topalian, S. L.,

Toy, S. T., Simon, P., Lotze, M. T., Yang, J. C., Seipp, C. A., Simpson, C., Carter, C., Bock, S., Schwartzentruber, D., Wei, J. P. and White, D. E. (1988). Use of tumor-infiltrating lymphocytes and interleukin-2 in the immunotherapy of patients with metastatic melanoma. A preliminary report. *New England Journal of Medicine*, **319**: 1676–80.

Rosenberg, S. A., Aebersold, P., Cornetta, K., Kasid, A., Morgan, R. A., Moen, R., Karson, E. M., Lotze, M. T., Yang, J. C., Topalian, S. L., Merino, M. J., Culver, K., Miller, A. D., Blaese, M. R. and Anderson, W. F. (1990a). Gene transfer into humans – immunotherapy of patients with advanced melanoma, using tumor-infiltrating lymphocytes modified by retroviral gene transduction. *New England Journal of Medicine*, **323**: 570–8.

Rosenberg, S. A., Blaese, R. M., Culver, K., Anderson, W. F., Cornetta, K. and Freeman, S. (1990b). The N2-TIL human gene transfer clinical protocol. *Human Gene Therapy*, **1**: 73–92.

Rosenberg, S. A., Kasid, A., Anderson, W. F., Blaese, R. M., Aebersold, P., Yang, J., Topalian, S., Kriegler, M., Maiorella, B., Moen, R. and Chiang, Y. (1990c). TNF/TIL human gene therapy clinical protocol. *Human Gene Therapy*, **1**: 443–62.

Rosenberg, S. A., Anderson, W. F., Asher, A. L., Blaese, M. R., Ettinghausen, S. E., Hwu, P., Kasid, A., Mule, J. J., Parkinson, D. R., Schwartzentruber, D. J., Topalian, S. L., Weber, J. S., Yannelli, J. R., Yang, J. C. and Linehan, W. M. (1992a). Immunization of cancer patients using autologous cancer cells modified by the insertion of the gene for tumor necrosis factor. *Human Gene Therapy*, **3**: 57–73.

Rosenberg, S. A., Anderson, W. F., Blaese, R. M., Ettinghausen, S. E., Hwu, P., Karp, S. E., Kasid, A., Mule, J. J., Parkinson, D. R., Salo, J. C., Schwartzentruber, D. J., Topalian, S. L., Weber, J. S., Yannelli, J. R., Yang, J. C. and Linehan, W. M. (1992b). Immunization of cancer patients using autologous cancer cells modified by the insertion of the gene for interleukin-2. *Human Gene Therapy*, **3**: 75–90.

The author thanks Billye Sanford of the Office of Recombinant DNA Activities, NIH, for providing numerous RAC documents.

10

Safety testing for gene therapy products

J. PATRICK CONDREAY

General considerations

In the USA the authority to regulate gene therapy products rests with the Center for Biologics Evaluation and Research (CBER) in the Food and Drug Administration (FDA). At present, all gene therapy products are at the investigational stage and are regulated under the standards for Investigational New Drugs (INDs) in 21 Code of Federal Regulations (CFR) part 312 (Taylor, 1993). Certain existing guidelines for the regulation of biologic therapeutics (21 CFR parts 210, 211, and 600) apply to the production of gene therapy products. Specifically, since biologicals cannot be completely defined, quality control on the starting materials and production process is equally as important as on the finished product to avoid the introduction of harmful contaminants. To outline the requirements for production of gene therapy products and to address issues that are more specific to the concerns unique to gene therapy approaches (e.g., genetic consequences), CBER has issued a series of 'Points to Consider' (PTC) documents to aid investigators with IND submissions.

Points to consider in human somatic cell therapy and gene therapy

At the time this document was drafted (Center for Biologics Evaluation and Research Staff, 1991) the majority of the protocols being submitted were ex-vivo cell therapies or cell-marking studies, thus its emphasis is on characterization of modified cell populations. Some of the concerns that are unique to gene therapy (as opposed to biologicals in general) are characterization of the genetic construct used as well as the vector system being used to transfer the construct, the method of its production, and verification that the vector does not replicate. Modified cells should be monitored for identity, loss of growth factor dependence, and their tumorigenicity as appropriate. Additionally, one should characterize the location, stability, and function of the genetic modification. Many of the concerns about the use of retroviral vectors as gene-transfer vectors for ex-vivo modification of cell populations are also relevant to the direct administration of viral vectors to patients (Epstein, 1991).

Supplement to the points to consider in the production and testing of new drugs and biologicals produced by recombinant DNA technology: nucleic acid characterization and genetic stability

The forerunner to this document was issued in 1985 (Center for Biologics Evaluation and Research Staff, 1985) and spelled out the biochemical characterization to be carried out on protein products. These guidelines (Center for Biologics Evaluation and Research Staff, 1993a) were issued to address the problems associated with detecting subtle changes in a product due to mutations in the expression construct. Many of these same concerns are applicable to genetic constructs and modified cell lines that are used to produce vectors for gene therapeutics. Complete characterization of the construct includes detailed descriptions of cloning and content, as well as a complete sequence. Once transferred into cells, the state of the insert and sequence of the relevant coding region must be determined for expression clones and master cell banks. Additionally, the same characterization should be done on one lot of 'end of production' cells.

Points to consider in the characterization of cell lines used to produce biologicals

This document (Center for Biologics Evaluation and Research Staff, 1993b) contains a fairly detailed outline of the quality control testing requirements for the establishment of production cell banks, validation of manufacturing processes, and safety of final product. Testing must be carried out following the guidelines for Good Laboratory Practice according to the 21 CFR part 58. The guidelines in this PTC are more specific than those in the document discussed above, since it addresses issues common to all biologicals and the safety considerations are better defined. Specific tests that are carried out on raw materials and cell lines will be discussed below.

Testing of raw materials

As mentioned above, quality control at all steps in bioprocessing is essential to avoid introducing contaminants during the process that must be removed or inactivated in the final product. This is of particular importance with respect to the raw materials used for cell culture media since cell propagation can amplify any agent present in the media. Quality control testing gets quite repetitive; many of the tests mentioned below need to be repeated at each step of the production process. If contaminants are detected in starting materials, it is possible that they can be eliminated by validated methods. However, if they are introduced late in the process, it might not be possible to treat the final material without affecting the product itself.

Production of therapeutics using cell substrates necessitates using products of animal origin, most commonly serum (or serum-derived factors) and trypsin. These materials must be tested according to protocols in 9 CFR part 113 and certified free of any adventitious agents. Most serum used in cell culture is of bovine origin and is tested for the presence of bovine viruses. This involves inoculating monolayers of Vero cells and bovine cells with test material and observing the cultures over several weeks, and subpassages for cytopathic effects (CPE); these cultures are eventually stained and examined for CPE. Subpassaging refers to the test cell monolayers and the supernatants from these cultures which are passaged on to fresh test cell monolayers. Certain viruses are noncytopathic and are detected by hemadsorption or staining with fluorescent antibodies against known viruses; for bovine material these are bovine viral diarrhea, bovine parvovirus, bovine adenoviruses, and rabies virus. The agent responsible for bovine spongiform encephalopathy (BSE) presents a problem since there is no test to detect it. Thus, the FDA requires the use of serum from countries that have been designated as free of BSE by the Department of Agriculture. Trypsin used for cell dissociation is generally of porcine origin, and similar tests must be performed on it using porcine indicator cells and antibodies to detect porcine viruses; these are transmissible gastroenteritis virus, porcine adenovirus, bovine diarrhea virus, and rabies virus.

Although bovine and porcine sources are the most common for media supplements, many growth factors are isolated from serum of other animals (e.g., human) or might be recombinant products produced in Chinese hamster ovary cells. The testing for adventitious viruses applies to any components expressed or isolated from a mammalian source and should be tailored for the appropriate species. Material derived from human sources should be tested for human retroviruses, Epstein–Barr virus, hepatitis B and C viruses, and cytomegalovirus. Material from rodent cell lines can be screened by antibody production tests in the appropriate species; this involves inoculating animals with test material and screening their serum for the production of antibodies directed against known agents.

Media components should also be tested for mycoplasmal contamination as spelled out in Attachment 2 to the PTC document on cell lines (Center for Biologics Evaluation and Research Staff, 1993b). There are three tests that are required for the detection of mycoplasma species. Test material is inoculated either on to agar plates and incubated under anaerobic conditions, or into a semisolid broth media which is incubated aerobically before subpassaging on to agar plates grown anaerobically. After several days of incubation, these cultures are examined for growth. In addition, material must be cultivated with Vero cells which are then stained with a fluorescent DNA-binding dye and examined for mycoplasma. Finally, media should be tested for sterility using the standards in 21 CFR part 610.12. This involves inoculating two types of media which are incubated for at least 14 days and examined throughout the incubation period for bacterial or fungal growth.

Cell/virus banks

To date, retrovirus and adenovirus are the only two viral vectors that have been used in gene therapy protocols (Crystal, 1995). While these two systems are quite different in the particulars of their production, and thus have specific safety considerations, both require the generation and characterization of cell banks following the guidelines of the PTC for cell lines (Center for Biologics Evaluation and Research Staff, 1993b) and PTC supplement on nucleic acid characterization (Center for Biologics Evaluation and Research Staff, 1993a). Testing need be carried out only once on cell banks. Cells to be used for production must be characterized as to their origin and history, and their identity by isoenzyme examination. The growth characteristics and particulars of cell propagation (e.g., media, doubling time, maximum passage number) must be fully described. Banks must be tested for sterility and mycoplasma as described above, as well as for the presence of adventitious agents specific to the origin and history of the cells (discussed below).

Cell banks for retroviral vectors

One of the major concerns for retroviral producer cells is the generation of replication competent retrovirus (RCR) through recombination between the construct containing the packaging functions, the therapeutic construct, or endogenous retroviral sequences. To detect the presence of RCR, amplification steps are carried out in *Mus dunni* cells by treating with culture supernatants from the producer cells and by coculturing the producer cells with the susceptible line. Supernatants from these amplification steps are then tested in a feline (PG4) S^+L^- focus assay to detect amphotropic and xenotropic retrovirus. There is a variety of assays that can be used to detect other murine retroviruses, such as the mouse (D56) S^+L^- focus assay, the XC syncytium formation assay, or an immunofluorescence assay on the infected *M. dunni* monolayers using a broad-spectrum antibody.

Further in-vitro and in-vivo testing must be done for adventitious virus that might be contaminating the cell bank, including the mouse antibody production test as outlined above. Material is examined in vitro by inoculating monolayers of human diploid cells, (e.g., MRC-5), Vero cells, and a cell line from the same species as the producer cell (generally murine). These cultures are examined for CPE and hemadsorption over a period of weeks, as described previously. Producer cell culture supernatants should also be injected into embryonated hen eggs, adult mice, and suckling mice, and the animals examined for evidence of viral pathogenicity.

Cell and virus banks for adenoviral vectors

Cell banks for adenovirus vector production require the same identity, sterility, mycoplasma, and bovine/porcine virus testing as outlined above. However, since the cells used for this purpose are of human origin (293 cells which express E1 gene functions), there are additional characterizations required. Tests for tumorigenicity of cells must be done using approved animal systems, though in-vitro assays (growth in soft agar) may be substituted if they can be demonstrated to be as sensitive as the in-vivo assays. The presence of human pathogenic viruses, such as hepatitis B and C, cytomegalovirus, and Epstein–Barr virus, must be tested for with in-vitro techniques. Human retroviruses are screened for by transmission electron microscopy of cells, as well as amplification techniques in susceptible cell populations followed by in-vitro detection of reverse transcriptase activity or polymerase chain reaction (PCR) detection. Certainly, a major concern would be the presence of replication competent adenovirus (RCA) in the culture supernatants of the cell substrate. These supernatants are inoculated on to monolayers of susceptible, non-E1-expressing cell lines (A549, Vero, HeLa) and the monolayers are examined for CPE, followed by passage of supernatants on to fresh monolayers as an amplification step (Wilson et al., 1994).

The production of adenoviral vectors requires the production of a master bank of the recombinant, defective virus which is subject to the same safety testing as the cell bank (sterility, adventitious viruses, etc.) and genetic characterization that is required for recombinant DNA products (description of construction, expression of therapeutic gene, genetic stability). These viral stocks must also be certified free of RCA. This can be done by the CPE assay described above, or with PCR assays designed to detect the deleted E1 regions in DNA isolated from the viral stock. The sensitivity of the PCR assay can be increased by amplification steps in susceptible cells which do not express the E1 helper functions. Functional tests for the recombinant vector would include infection of a susceptible cell line followed by detection of the therapeutic gene product in the infected cell.

Cell banks for plasmid production

Cell banks of *E. coli* for the production of plasmid DNA for gene transfer are subject to similar standards of identity and purity (i.e., auxotrophic markers, freedom from fungi, etc.) that are required for mammalian cells. Cells, plasmid constructs, and methods of handling need to be described and characterized according to the PTC documents (Center for Biologics Evaluation and Research Staff, 1993a, 1993b). Genetic stability of the plasmid and functionality of the therapeutic gene must also be demonstrated. An additional concern about the production of plasmid DNA in bacteria is the use of penicillin-type antibiotics in fermentation runs due to the possibility of inducing hypersensitivy in patients (Center for Biologics Evaluation and Research Staff, 1985).

Final product testing

Production lots of gene therapy vectors must be put through the same sterility and mycoplasma tests that have been described previously; additionally, the stability and functionality of the vector and therapeutic construct must be tested in a product-specific manner. A general safety test as described in 21 CFR 610.11 must be carried out; this involves injection of the product into rodents followed by monitoring of animals for weight loss or toxicity. Some of the standards for purity which are mentioned in the PTC (Center for Biologics Evaluation and Research Staff, 1993b) are that residual serum should not exceed 1 ppm, and that DNA from the cell substrate used to produce the vector should be 100 pg/dose or less. Endotoxin content is a concern for all vectors, especially plasmid constructs which are produced in bacterial hosts; the Limulus Amebocyte Lysate test is used to evaluate samples. For viral vectors, one must obviously assay for infectious titer of the recombinant vector (since this is related to dose) as well as test for the presence of replication competent helper virus. However, there are some concerns specific to the two different viral systems. Adenovirus vectors must be assayed for total particle density (by ultraviolet absorbance, light scattering, or electron microscopy) as well as infectious unit density since defective vectors are capable of inducing toxic effects. In the case of retroviral vectors, end of production cells must be recovered and tested for RCR breakouts.

Patient concerns

Concerns about patient safety and monitoring are fairly specific to the individual treatment regimen that is being proposed, and thus must be assessed on a case-by-case basis. However, there are some general concerns for gene therapy approaches. Researchers should be prepared to address possible toxic effects due to gene delivery to sites other than the intended site, or the immunogenicity of the therapeutic gene product. A particular concern in using adenoviral vectors is the inflammatory response seen in human subjects which was not predicted by animal models (Crystal, 1995). The major toxicity concern about retroviruses stems from toxicity of RCR demonstrated in immunosuppressed primates, and the FDA requires periodic, long-term monitoring of patients treated with retroviral vectors for RCR infection (Woodcock, 1993).

Conclusion

The recommendations outlined above are general guidelines for safety concerns with respect to gene therapy products. The FDA considers each biologic therapy as a unique entity and encourages investigators to work interactively with regulators to establish exact IND requirements for an individual product (Kessler et al., 1993). Furthermore, the FDA realizes that gene therapy is an evolving field, and that new safety concerns will emerge as the field matures and more data are collected (Epstein, 1991).

References

Center for Biologics Evaluation and Research Staff (1985). *Points to Consider in the Production and Testing of New Drugs and Biologicals Produced by Recombinant DNA Technology.* Congressional and Consumer Affairs Branch, Food and Drug Administration, Washington DC.
Center for Biologics Evaluation and Research Staff (1991). Points to consider in

human somatic cell therapy and gene therapy. *Human Gene Therapy*, **2**: 251–6.

Center for Biologics Evaluation and Research Staff (1993a). Supplement to the points to consider in the production and testing of new drugs and biologicals produced by recombinant DNA technology: Nucleic acid characterization and genetic stability. *Biologics*, **21**: 81–3.

Center for Biologics Evaluation and Research Staff (1993b). *Points to Consider in the Characterization of Cell Lines Used to Produce Biologicals*. Congressional and Consumer Affairs Branch, Food and Drug Administration, Washington DC.

Crystal, R. G. (1995). Transfer of genes to humans: early lessons and obstacles to success. *Science*, **270**: 404–10.

Epstein, S. L. (1991). Regulatory concerns in human gene therapy. *Human Gene Therapy*, **2**: 243–9.

Kessler, D. A., Siegel, J. P., Noguchi, P. D., Zoon, K. C., Feiden, K. L. and Woodcock, J. (1993). Regulation of somatic-cell therapy and gene therapy by the Food and Drug Administration. *New England Journal of Medicine*, **329**: 1169–73.

Taylor, M. R. (1993). Application of current statutory authorities to human somatic cell therapy products and gene therapy products. *Federal Register*, **58**: 53248–51.

Wilson, J. M., Engelhardt, J. F., Grossman, M., Simon, R. H. and Yang, Y. (1994). Gene therapy of cystic fibrosis lung disease using E1 deleted adenoviruses: a phase I trial. *Human Gene Therapy*, **5**: 501–19.

Woodcock, J. (1993). *Letter to sponsors of INDs using a retroviral vector*. Congressional and Consumer Affairs Branch, Food and Drug Administration, Washington DC.

Index